Vasculitis in Rheumatic Diseases

Editor

DANIEL A. ALBERT

RHEUMATIC DISEASE CLINICS OF NORTH AMERICA

www.rheumatic.theclinics.com

Consulting Editor
MICHAEL H. WEISMAN

February 2015 • Volume 41 • Number 1

ELSEVIER

1600 John F. Kennedy Boulevard • Suite 1800 • Philadelphia, Pennsylvania, 19103-2899
http://www.theclinics.com

RHEUMATIC DISEASE CLINICS OF NORTH AMERICA Volume 41, Number 1
February 2015 ISSN 0889-857X, ISBN 13: 978-0-323-35450-9

Editor: Jennifer Flynn-Briggs
Developmental Editor: Casey Jackson

Rheumatic Disease Clinics of North America (ISSN 0889-857X) is published quarterly by Elsevier Inc., 360 Park Avenue South, New York, NY 10010-1710. Months of issue are February, May, August, and November. Business and editorial offices: 1600 John F. Kennedy Boulevard, Suite 1800, Philadelphia, PA 19103-2899. Periodicals postage paid at New York, NY and additional mailing offices. Subscription prices are USD 335.00 per year for US individuals, USD 579.00 per year for US institutions, USD 165.00 per year for US students and residents, USD 395.00 per year for Canadian individuals, USD 722.00 per year for Canadian institutions, USD 465.00 per year for international individuals, USD 722.00 per year for international institutions, and USD 230.00 per year for Canadian and foreign students/residents. To receive student/resident rate, orders must be accompanied by name of affiliated institution, date of term, and the *signature* of program/residency coordinator on institution letterhead. Orders will be billed at individual rate until proof of status received. Foreign air speed delivery is included in all *Clinics* subscription prices. All prices are subject to change without notice. **POSTMASTER:** Send address changes to *Rheumatic Disease Clinics of North America,* Elsevier Health Sciences Division, Subscription Customer Service, 3251 Riverport Lane, Maryland Heights, MO 63043. **Customer Service: 1-800-654-2452 (US and Canada). From outside of the US and Canada: 314-447-8871. Fax: 314-447-8029. For print support, e-mail: JournalsCustomerService-usa@elsevier.com. For online support, e-mail: JournalsOnline Support-usa@elsevier.com.**

Reprints. For copies of 100 or more of articles in this publication, please contact the Commercial Reprints Department, Elsevier Inc., 360 Park Avenue South, New York, New York, 10010-1710; Tel.: +1-212-633-3874, Fax: +1-212-633-3820, and E-mail: reprints@elsevier.com.

Rheumatic Disease Clinics of North America is covered in *MEDLINE/PubMed (Index Medicus), Current Contents/Clinical Medicine, Science Citation Index, ISI/BIOMED,* and *EMBASE/Excerpta Medica.*

Contributors

CONSULTING EDITOR

MICHAEL H. WEISMAN, MD
Professor of Medicine, Division of Rheumatology, Cedars-Sinai Medical Center,
Los Angeles, California

EDITOR

DANIEL A. ALBERT, MD
Professor of Medicine and Pediatrics, Dartmouth-Hitchcock Medical Center, The Geisel
School of Medicine at Dartmouth and The Dartmouth Institute, Lebanon, New Hampshire

AUTHORS

MARCO A. ALBA, MD
Vasculitis Research Unit, Department of Systemic Autoimmune Diseases, Hospital
Clínic, Institut d'Investigacions Biomèdiques August Pi i Sunyer (IDIBAPS), Barcelona,
Spain

SERGUEI BANNYKH, MD, PhD
Department of Pathology, Cedars-Sinai Medical Center, Los Angeles, California

MARIA C. CID, MD
Vasculitis Research Unit, Department of Systemic Autoimmune Diseases, Hospital
Clínic, Institut d'Investigacions Biomèdiques August Pi i Sunyer (IDIBAPS), University
of Barcelona, Barcelona, Spain

GEORGINA ESPÍGOL-FRIGOLÉ, MD
Vasculitis Research Unit, Department of Systemic Autoimmune Diseases, Hospital
Clínic, Institut d'Investigacions Biomèdiques August Pi i Sunyer (IDIBAPS), Barcelona,
Spain

LINDSY FORBESS, MD, MSc
Clinical Instructor of Medicine, Department of Rheumatology, Cedars-Sinai Medical
Center, Los Angeles, California

ANA GARCÍA-MARTÍNEZ, MD
Vasculitis Research Unit, Emergency Department, Hospital Clínic, Institut d'Investigacions
Biomèdiques August Pi i Sunyer (IDIBAPS), Barcelona, Spain

ROSA GILABERT, MD
Center for Diagnostic Imaging, Hospital Clínic, Institut d'Investigacions Biomèdiques
August Pi i Sunyer (IDIBAPS), University of Barcelona, Barcelona, Spain

DANIELA GHETIE, MD
Division of Arthritis & Rheumatic Diseases, Vasculitis Center, Oregon Health & Science
University, Portland, Oregon

JOSÉ HERNÁNDEZ-RODRÍGUEZ, MD
Vasculitis Research Unit, Department of Systemic Autoimmune Diseases, Hospital Clínic, Institut d'Investigacions Biomèdiques August Pi i Sunyer (IDIBAPS), University of Barcelona, Barcelona, Spain

LINDSAY LALLY, MD
Division of Rheumatology, Hospital for Special Surgery, New York, New York

NAVID MEHRABAN, MD
Division of Arthritis & Rheumatic Diseases, Vasculitis Center, Oregon Health & Science University, Portland, Oregon

ROBERT G. MICHELETTI, MD
Assistant Professor of Dermatology and Medicine, Perelman School of Medicine at the University of Pennsylvania, Philadelphia, Pennsylvania

ELI M. MILOSLAVSKY, MD
Instructor in Medicine, Harvard Medical School, Rheumatology Unit, Massachusetts General Hospital, Boston, Massachusetts

PAUL A. MONACH, MD, PhD
Vasculitis Center, Section of Rheumatology, Department of Medicine, Boston University School of Medicine, Boston, Massachusetts

SERGIO PRIETO-GONZÁLEZ, MD
Vasculitis Research Unit, Department of Systemic Autoimmune Diseases, Hospital Clínic, Institut d'Investigacions Biomèdiques August Pi i Sunyer (IDIBAPS), Barcelona, Spain

ALICIA RODRIGUEZ-PLA, MD, PhD, MPH
Section of Rheumatology, Department of Medicine, Boston University School of Medicine, Boston, Massachusetts

LISA R. SAMMARITANO, MD
Division of Rheumatology, Hospital for Special Surgery, New York, New York

CAILIN H. SIBLEY, MD, MHS
Division of Arthritis & Rheumatic Diseases, Vasculitis Center, Oregon Health & Science University, Portland, Oregon

ORA SINGER, MD, MS
Division of Rheumatology, University of Michigan, Ann Arbor, Michigan

ROBERT SPIERA, MD
Division of Rheumatology, Hospital for Special Surgery, New York, New York

JOHN H. STONE, MD, MPH
Professor of Medicine, Harvard Medical School, Rheumatology Unit, Massachusetts General Hospital, Boston, Massachusetts

ROBERT P. SUNDEL, MD
Director of Rheumatology, Boston Children's Hospital, Associate Professor of Pediatrics, Harvard Medical School, Boston, Massachusetts

ITZIAR TAVERA-BAHILLO, MD
Vasculitis Research Unit, Department of Systemic Autoimmune Diseases, Hospital Clínic, Institut d'Investigacions Biomèdiques August Pi i Sunyer (IDIBAPS), Barcelona, Spain

SEBASTIAN H. UNIZONY, MD
Instructor in Medicine, Harvard Medical School, Rheumatology Unit, Massachusetts General Hospital, Boston, Massachusetts

VICTORIA P. WERTH, MD
Professor of Dermatology and Medicine, Philadelphia Veterans Affairs Medical Center, Perelman School of Medicine at the University of Pennsylvania, Philadelphia, Pennsylvania

Contents

This article provides an update on the diagnosis and management of the antineutrophil cytoplasmic antibody (ANCA)-associated vasculitides, granulomatosis with polyangiitis (formerly Wegener), microscopic polyangiitis, and eosinophilic granulomatosis with polyangiitis (formerly Churg-Strauss). Focus is on new schemes of classification and the importance of ANCAs in the diagnosis and prognosis of these systemic vasculitides. Current therapeutic strategies consisting of glucocorticoids in conjunction with conventional or biologic agents for both induction of remission and remission maintenance are outlined. Future research directions include investigation of the optimal duration and frequency of maintenance therapy and development of targeted therapeutic agents.

Small vessel vasculitis in the skin manifests with palpable purpura on the lower extremities. This clinical presentation prompts a complete physical examination, history, and review of systems, as well as biopsies for routine processing and direct immunofluorescence to confirm the diagnosis. The presence of vasculitis in other organs, associated underlying conditions, and the severity of cutaneous manifestations dictate management. The majority of cases are self-limited, and overall the prognosis is favorable. Still, a subset of patients can have serious complications and chronic or recurrent disease.

Polyarteritis nodosa (PAN) is a systemic disease, but variants are cutaneous PAN and single-organ disease. Histologic confirmation of vasculitis in medium-sized arteries is desirable, and biopsies should be obtained from the symptomatic and least invasive sites. Angiography can show multiple microaneurysms in the viscera. Treatment includes high-dose corticosteroids, which are combined with immunosuppressive agents when internal organs are involved and with life-threatening disease. Once remission is achieved, maintenance agents are initiated. PAN is becoming a rare disease. International collaborative efforts are under way to establish better diagnostic and classification for all vasculitides, including PAN.

Primary angiitis of the central nervous system (PACNS) is a rare disease, although it is increasingly recognized both in adults and children. Little is known about pathogenesis, but efforts at classification into subtypes are being made, and the distinction of PACNS from reversible cerebral vasoconstriction syndrome has been a major advance. The prognosis for improvement, or at least stabilization, of neurologic function is good with prompt and aggressive treatment, but the diagnosis continues to be challenging. Refinement of treatment strategies is needed. Multicenter collaboration may be crucial to make additional progress via randomized trials.

Kawasaki disease (KD) is the archetypal pediatric vasculitis, exemplifying the unique aspects and challenges of vascular inflammation in children. The condition is almost unheard of in adults, is closely associated with infections, and is self-limited, with fever resolving after an average of 12 days even without treatment. Yet KD is also a potentially fatal disease and the most common cause of acquired heart disease in the developed world. Unraveling of the developmental, immunologic, and genetic secrets of Kawasaki disease promises to improve our understanding of vasculitis in particular, and perhaps also to provide a window on the fundamental mysteries of inflammatory diseases in general.

Cogan and Behcet syndromes are considered large vessel vasculitides. Both are rare diseases, with varied clinical manifestations affecting multiple organ systems. Although both have hallmark symptoms (ocular and vestibuloauditory inflammation in Cogan syndrome and aphthous ulcers in Behcet syndrome), neither has confirmatory diagnostic testing. Delayed diagnosis can result in poor outcomes. In both syndromes, large vessel arterial inflammation may result in severe morbidity and mortality. Treatment strategies in both syndromes vary based on organ system involvement and severity of manifestations. In this article, the epidemiology, proposed pathogenesis, manifestations, and the most current treatment paradigms for these syndromes are reviewed.

Cryoglobulins are immunoglobulins that precipitate at temperatures less than 37°C. They occur secondary to infectious, autoimmune, and malignant processes. In the Brouet classification, type I cryoglobulinemia is caused by hyperviscosity, whereas type II and III manifestations are caused by vasculitis in target organs (primarily skin, peripheral nerves, and kidney). New classification criteria were recently proposed that may help with study and treatment of cryoglobulinemic vasculitis (CryoVas).

Hepatitis C virus is the most common cause of CryoVas and treatment with antivirals can be curative in mild cases, whereas rituximab is highly effective in treating active vasculitis in more severe cases.

The major manifestations of antiphospholipid syndrome (APS) are caused by thrombosis within the venous or arterial vasculature, whereas the vascular lesions in systemic vasculitis result from an inflammatory infiltrate in the vessel wall. There is an association between vascular thrombosis and inflammation, however, as vasculitis can occur in APS and thromboembolic complications are seen in systemic vasculitis. Although differentiating between vasculitis and antiphospholipid-associated thrombosis can be difficult, it may be crucial to do so given the different therapeutic implications for immunosuppression or anticoagulation. This article explores the relationship between thrombosis and inflammation as it relates to APS and systemic vasculitis.

The diagnosis of large-vessel vasculitis has experienced substantial improvement in recent years. While Takayasu arteritis diagnosis relies on imaging, the involvement of epicranial arteries by giant-cell arteritis facilitates histopathological confirmation. When appropriately performed temporal artery biopsy has high sensitivity and specificity. However, an optimal biopsy is not always achievable and, occasionally, the superficial temporal artery may not be involved. Imaging in its various modalities including colour-duplex ultrasonography, computed tomography angiography, magnetic resonance angiography and positron emission tomography, are emerging as important procedures for the diagnosis and assessment of disease extent in large-vessel vasculitis. Recent contributions to the better performance and interpretation of temporal artery biopsies as well as advances in imaging are the focus of the present review.

The need to distinguish true primary systemic vasculitis from its multiple potential mimickers is one of the most challenging diagnostic conundrums in clinical medicine. This article reviews 9 challenging vasculitis mimickers: fibromuscular dysplasia, calciphylaxis, segmental arterial mediolysis, antiphospholipid syndrome, hypereosinophilic syndrome, lymphomatoid granulomatosis, malignant atrophic papulosis, livedoid vasculopathy, and immunoglobulin G4–related disease.

RHEUMATIC DISEASE CLINICS OF NORTH AMERICA

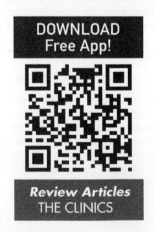

Foreword

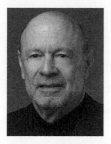

Michael H. Weisman, MD
Consulting Editor

Dan Albert has assembled an outstanding collection of articles that not only depict the latest advances in diagnosis and management of various forms of vasculitis but also touch on emerging issues of epidemiology, genetics, and environmental triggers. Where there is clinical trial evidence for management approaches, this is highlighted and emphasized. The focus of these articles is clinical and practical—reserving in-depth discussion of possible pathogenenic mechanisms to larger textbooks, but with references abounding in our issue. These conditions always present diagnostic dilemmas and challenges because neither pathology, laboratory investigations, nor signs and symptoms provide sufficient specificity for a cookbook or algorithm approach. Perhaps it is this challenge that makes rheumatologists experts in these conditions and might even provide a motivation for many to go into the field in the first place. There can be no one more suited to fit these criteria than Dr Albert himself—a superb clinician with a scholarly mind and an analytic approach to everything he does. We are very proud of this volume.

Michael H. Weisman, MD
Division of Rheumatology
Cedars-Sinai Medical Center
8700 Beverly Boulevard
Los Angeles, CA 90024, USA

E-mail address:
michael.weisman@cshs.org

Rheum Dis Clin N Am 41 (2015) xi
http://dx.doi.org/10.1016/j.rdc.2014.10.002
0889-857X/15/$ – see front matter © 2015 Published by Elsevier Inc.

rheumatic.theclinics.com

Preface

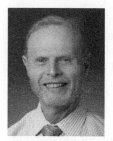

Daniel A. Albert, MD
Editor

Book length treatises on Vasculitis are uncommon but necessary for practicing rheumatologists, who are unlikely to see patients with these disorders frequently enough to be familiar with all the nuances of their presentation and management. We have assembled an outstanding group of experts to present a clinically comprehensive but concise and current summary of each of the major vasculitic syndromes. While the etiology of most of these conditions remains elusive, the diagnosis and treatment have progressed rapidly, and we are pleased to acknowledge that these articles represent state-of-the-art management advice.

This issue covers the spectrum from small to large vessel and from relatively common to excruciatingly rare disorders. In some areas, the progress has been dramatic, as detailed in the superb article by Spiera and colleagues on GPA, MPA, and EGPA. Other areas are more slowly evolving, such as small-vessel vasculitis, which straddles the boundary between rheumatology and dermatology as the authors Werth and Micheletti do in real life. Some of the disorders seem to be increasing in recognition (if not frequency), like GPA, and others are disappearing, as Drs Forbess and Bannykh detail in an article on polyarteritis nodosa, which is so rarely seen that rheumatologists often have no first-hand experience with it.

Central nervous system vasculitis has become much more complex, as Drs Rodriguez-Pla and Monach point out, with the recognition of vasospastic disorders that are sometimes difficult to discriminate from inflammatory syndromes.

Kawasaki disease is much more common in Asia than in the United States, but Dr Sundel at Boston Children's Hospital has an unusually broad experience and has published important articles on the topic.

Cogan and Behcet disease are among the least common of the vasculitides, and cases are often directed to centers with neuro-ophthalmology and neuro-otology departments. These pleomorphic conditions are ably reviewed by Dr Singer from the University of Michigan.

Cryoglobulinemia is common in countries with a high prevalence of hepatitis C but may become less common, as PAN did, with the introduction of therapy that eradicates the viral infection. Dr Sibley and colleagues present a comprehensive summary of this topic.

Rheum Dis Clin N Am 41 (2015) xiii–xiv
http://dx.doi.org/10.1016/j.rdc.2014.10.003
0889-857X/15/$ – see front matter © 2015 Elsevier Inc. All rights reserved.

rheumatic.theclinics.com

Antiphospholipid syndrome can mimic many inflammatory vasculitides. Drs Lally and Sammartino report on our progress in understanding this syndrome from a center that specializes in this condition at Cornell Medical Center in New York.

Large-vessel vasculitis encompasses one of the most common vasculidites (giant cell arteritis) and one of the least common (Takayasu), which, although separated by the age of the patient, occasionally are difficult to distinguish. Dr Cid and colleagues are leaders in the field of large-vessel vasculitis diagnosis and review that topic in detail.

Last, one of the leaders in the field, Dr Stone, and his colleagues review the range of mimics that can fool even experienced rheumatologists. This is a crucial issue for practicing rheumatologists.

All in all, even experts will find ample new material and guidance for the management of these difficult syndromes.

Daniel A. Albert, MD
Geisel School of Medicine, Dartmouth
Dartmouth-Hitchcock Medical Center
Rheumatology
One Medical Center Drive
Lebanon, NH 03756, USA

E-mail address:
daniel.a.albert@hitchcock.org

Current Landscape of Antineutrophil Cytoplasmic Antibody-Associated Vasculitis

Classification, Diagnosis, and Treatment

Lindsay Lally, MD*, Robert Spiera, MD

KEYWORDS

- ANCA-associated vasculitis • Granulomatosis with polyangiitis (Wegener)
- Microscopic polyangiitis
- Eosinophilic granulomatosis with polyangiitis (Churg-Strauss)

KEY POINTS

- Antineutrophil cytoplasmic antibody (ANCA) positivity by immunofluorescence should be confirmed with ELISA for proteinase-3 (PR3) or myeloperoxidase (MPO) in the diagnosis of ANCA-associated vasculitides (AAVs). Tissue biopsy for histologic confirmation should be obtained whenever possible.
- ANCA specificity may be associated with different prognostic and phenotypic features in granulomatosis with polyangiitis (GPA) and microscopic polyangiitis (MPA). Additionally, in eosinophilic granulomatosis with polyangiitis (EGPA), different clinical manifestations may be observed in those with ANCA positivity compared with those who are ANCA negative.
- Treatment of AAVs, which is divided into an induction phase followed by remission maintenance, should be tailored to disease activity and severity. Optimal duration of maintenance therapy is unknown.

INTRODUCTION

The AAVs include GPA, formerly Wegener's granulomatosis; MPA; and EGPA, formerly Churg-Strauss syndrome. These 3 primary systemic vasculitides are multisystem diseases characterized by pauci-immune necrotizing vasculitis of small- to

Disclosure Statement: The authors have nothing to disclose.
Division of Rheumatology, Hospital for Special Surgery, 535 East 70th Street, New York, NY 10021, USA
* Corresponding author.
E-mail address: lallyl@hss.edu

medium-sized blood vessels and an association with serologically detectable ANCAs in a majority of cases. Change has transformed the field of AAVs in recent years with the introduction of new nomenclature for these diseases, novel insights into the genetic underpinnings of AAVs, and advances in therapeutic approach, including the use of biologics.[1–4] This article focuses on the current understanding of AAV diagnosis and management and highlights existing controversies and unmet needs in the care of patients with AAVs. Because of differences in clinical phenotype, disease course, and serologic positivity, EGPA is discussed separately at the end of this article.

CLASSIFICATION AND NOMENCLATURE

The 1990 American College of Rheumatology (ACR) classification criteria for the systemic vasculitides proposed a series of criteria meant to enable discrimination between the various forms of systemic vasculitis.[5,6] At the time the ACR criteria were created, MPA was not recognized as a distinct entity; thus, classification criteria for MPA were not created. As such, the ACR criteria for GPA are of limited value in differentiating between GPA and MPA. These classification criteria were created before ANCA testing was widely available, so ANCAs, which have an undisputed role in the diagnosis of AAVs, were excluded from classification criteria.

Despite high sensitivity and specificity, ACR criteria are of limited value in AAVs, especially in distinguishing between GPA and MPA, which have certain clinical and histologic differences. GPA is characterized by necrotizing small vessel vasculitis with extravascular granulomatous inflammation, which is not present in MPA. Although pulmonary and renal involvement is common in both GPA and MPA, granulomatous involvement of the upper and lower airway occurs exclusively in GPA. Otolaryngologic manifestations, including rhinosinusitis, serous otitis media, and subglottic inflammation, are present in an estimated 90% of patients with GPA, making this the most commonly involved organ system in GPA,[7] whereas glomerulonephritis is the most frequent manifestation in MPA. These phenotypic distinctions may confer important prognostic and therapeutic differences, discussed later.

In 2012, the International Chapel Hill Consensus Conference on the Nomenclature of Systemic Vasculitides (CHCC) was convened with a goal of redefining the vasculitic syndromes with nomenclature reflective of the underlying pathogenesis, pathology, and clinical characteristics.[1] The 2012 CHCC nosology eliminated eponyms from the AAV nomenclature and cemented presence of granulomatous inflammation in the respiratory tract as the key difference between GPA and MPA. This nomenclature fails to account for ANCA antigen specificity, which some experts think should be included with clinicopathologic phenotype in classification of AAVs.[8,9] Efforts to create more comprehensive classification and diagnostic criteria for AAV are under way with an international observational study designed to develop and validate classification and diagnostic criteria for primary systemic vasculitis, including the AAVs.[10]

ANTINEUTROPHIL CYTOPLASMIC ANTIBODY
Antineutrophil Cytoplasmic Antibody Detection

Circulating ANCAs with different immunofluorescence patterns and antigen specificities characterize GPA and MPA. ANCAs, which have demonstrated pathogenicity in animal, in vitro, and ex vivo models,[11,12] are also an important diagnostic tool. In making a diagnosis of AAVs, the utility of ANCAs depends on the clinical setting and on the assay used. A perinuclear (p-ANCA) or cytoplasmic (c-ANCA) pattern may be seen by indirect immunofluorescence; however, this technique is hampered by potential for interference by antinuclear antibodies and subjective interpretation. Positive immunofluorescence should be followed by ELISA for ANCAs specifically directed against PR3 or MPO, which are associated with GPA and MPA, respectively, in greater than 80% of cases.[13,14] New methodology for autoantigen detection, including new-generation ELISA and multiplex technology, will improve ANCA detection in the future.[15] C-ANCA pattern with PR3 positivity can be found in 90% of patients with active GPA,[13] and a majority of MPA patients have p-ANCA with positive MPO.[14] In the appropriate clinical setting, only combinations of c-ANCA with PR3 or p-ANCA with MPO have a positive predictive value for diagnosis of GPA or MPA.[16]

An atypical ANCA pattern on immunofluorescence, multiple positive autoantigens, or discordance between ANCA pattern and antigen specificity should alert suspicion for drug-induced disease, in particular cocaine. The most common autoantibody in cocaine-induced disease, which can mimic the destructive sinonasal disease of GPA, is directed against human neutrophil elastase.[17] This atypical ANCA is not found in patients with AAVs.

The clinical and pathogenic significance of additional ANCAs, other than the commercially available PR3 and MPO, are under investigation in AAVs. One such auto-antibody is human lysosomal-associated membrane protein 2 (LAMP-2). LAMP-2 is coexpressed with MPO and PR3 in neutrophils; however, unlike MPO and PR3, LAMP-2 is also expressed in glomerular endothelial cells, a key site of injury in AAVs. LAMP-2 autoantibodies were initially reported to be present in 85% of patients with untreated AAVs,[18] a finding that was duplicated by the same investigators in a different cohort of AAV patients with glomerulonephritis where LAMP-2 positivity was specific for AAVs and paralleled disease activity.[19] Another group found LAMP-2 in only 20% of AAV patients, however, which approached the frequency in their control population.[20] Given these conflicting results and lack of commercial grade assays, the value of LAMP-2 detection in AAVs remains unknown.

Implications of Antineutrophil Cytoplasmic Antibody Specificity

There has been increasing appreciation of phenotypic distinction between AAV patients with PR3 and MPO positivity. A recent genome-wide association study identified distinct genetic subsets of AAV patients, determined by ANCA antigen specificity and not clinical syndrome; different HLA correlations were noted in those with PR3-ANCA and MPO-ANCA.[2] Additionally, PR3 positivity was associated with genes coding for PR3 and α_1-antitrypsin. Exploring these genetic associations may allow for better appreciation of distinctions between disease pathogenesis depending on autoantigen subtype and possibly provide a platform for future genetic markers to aid diagnosis.

Prognostic differences between PR3 and MPO positivity also exist. Compared with MPO-ANCA, PR3-ANCA is associated with a higher mortality (relative risk >3).[21] Additional studies have identified PR3 positivity as an independent predictor of disease relapse.[22] In a cohort of more than 500 patients with AAVs and biopsy-proved glomerulonephritis, PR3 specificity conferred a 2-fold risk for relapse compared with MPO.[23] ANCA specificity for PR3 was independently associated with relapse regardless of pathology or clinical classification using the CHCC definitions of AAVs. Those with PR3-ANCA and renal disease may also have a faster decline in renal function compared with MPO-ANCA patients, although these data reflect deterioration prior to initiation of treatment.[24] A recent cluster analysis of approximately 700 patients enrolled in AAV treatment trials identified 5 subgroups of AAV patients based on several clinical variables and ANCA specificity.[25] Two of these subgroups were defined by renal involvement with or without PR3 positivity; patients in the renal

AAVs with PR3 subgroup had higher relapse risk but lower mortality rate than those with renal disease and no PR3.

Serial Antineutrophil Cytoplasmic Antibody Measurements and Correlation with Disease Activity

Although ANCA detection has diagnostic and prognostic importance in AAVs, the utility of serial ANCA measurements is less certain. Considerable variability exists in the available literature addressing the value of serial ANCAs, with differences in ANCA detection methodology, follow-up intervals, and definitions of disease activity, which makes drawing definitive conclusions difficult.[26–29] Observational cohorts have failed to show a definitive correlation between ANCA levels and disease activity or flare. A longitudinal analysis of 156 GPA patients participating in the Wegener's Granulomatosis Etanercept Trial (WGET) showed that changes in ANCAs accounted for less than 10% of changes in disease activity; relapse within 1 year of increasing PR3 titer was seen in only 40% of patients.[26]

A 2012 meta-analysis examining the value of serial ANCA measurements during remission to predict relapse included 18 articles looking at patients with either rising ANCA titer or persistently positive ANCAs.[28] Trying to account for heterogeneity between studies, the investigators found that rising ANCAs or persistently positive ANCAs was associated with flare (positive likelihood ratios 2.84 and 1.97, respectively); however, they concluded that ANCA titer alone was insufficient to guide treatment decisions. Persistently negative ANCAs in a patient who was previously ANCA positive do not guarantee disease quiescence. In a study of 100 AAV patients followed prospectively with serial ANCAs, 13 of the 37 patients who relapsed were ANCA negative at time of relapse.[29] In the right clinical setting and with supporting pathology when available, ANCAs remain a cornerstone for AAV diagnosis but are insufficiently sensitive or specific for monitoring disease activity, predicting relapse, or guiding immunosuppressive treatment. On an individual level, in patients in whom a relationship between ANCA level and disease activity has been established, serial ANCA testing may have a role in disease monitoring and therapeutic decision making.[16]

TISSUE BIOPSY

Guided tissue biopsies are important in defining the character and extent of the inflammatory process in the diagnosis of AAVs. Histologic confirmation of AAVs with tissue biopsy should be attempted whenever possible, but treatment should not be delayed in a critically ill patient with high suspicion for disease in whom tissue is not readily or safely accessible. Individual clinical presentation should dictate the biopsy location with the overall aim of performing the safest procedure with the highest potential yield.[30] Diagnostic yield varies depending on organ system biopsied, especially because inflammatory changes may be patchy and examination of large amount of tissue may be required to make a histopathologic diagnosis. In conjunction with clinical and serologic information, histologic evidence of necrotizing vasculitis with accompanying granulomatous inflammation is used to differentiate GPA from MPA.

Although upper airway disease is noted in three-quarters of GPA patients at disease onset, tissue biopsy of these regions has low yield for identifying the classical pathologic necrotizing vasculitis with granulomatous inflammation. One study noted necrotizing vasculitis with concurrent extravascular granulomatosis in only 16% of upper airway biopsies.[31] Other studies have found diagnostic yield of minimally invasive endonasal biopsy to approach 50%, especially in early or localized ENT disease, although this depends on location, depth, and number of samples biopsied.[32,33] In routine practice, however, even when performed by an experienced surgeon, upper airway biopsy is rarely diagnostic.

In patients with evidence of renal involvement based on urinalysis or reduced creatinine clearance, kidney biopsy remains the gold standard for diagnosis of glomerulonephritis. Kidney biopsy has a high yield with varying degrees of segmental necrotizing pauci-immune glomerulonephritis in greater than 80% of specimens.[34] Renal histopathology also has prognostic implications, according to a 2010 classification system of glomerular lesions,[35] with sclerosis and tubular atrophy correlated with progression to end-stage renal disease.[36]

Pulmonary involvement occurs in approximately 85% of AAV patients.[7] Pulmonary lesions in GPA are commonly nodules and cavitary changes whereas MPA patients present more frequently with pulmonary infiltrates or diffuse alveolar hemorrhage. Targeted biopsy of radiographically abnormal lung parenchyma via a thoracoscopic or open lung biopsy is usually of high yield for AAV diagnosis. The efficacy of transbronchial biopsy, however, in establishing the diagnosis of pulmonary vasculitis is less than 10%, and a negative transbronchial specimen should not exclude the diagnosis of AAVs.[37] Transbronchial specimens can be used to exclude infection or neoplasia, and bronchial alveolar lavage is helpful in confirming alveolar hemorrhage.

TREATMENT
Historical Perspective

The past several decades have seen major therapeutic advances in the management of AAVs. Primarily, recognition that a regimen of daily oral cyclophosphamide (CYC) and high-dose corticosteroids was effective for inducing remission in a vast majority of patients transformed AAVs from a uniformly fatal disease to a chronic relapsing disease with a dramatically reduced mortality of 25% at 5 years.[38] Although the initial observational data supporting the use of CYC reflects the experience of physicians at the National Institutes of Health caring for a cohort of GPA patients,[7] similar trends are evident in MPA. Progress has also been made in identification of various immunosuppressive agents with more favorable safety profiles than CYC, which can be used maintain remission; multiple randomized trials comparing maintenance regimens are discussed later (**Table 1**). In an effort to minimize toxicity related to CYC, there was the additional insight that some patients could be successfully treated with CYC-free regimens.[39] The past decade has seen the last major advance in AAV treatment born out of the search for more targeted therapy, with multicenter collaborations investigating the use of various biologic therapies.[3,4,40] Targeting of B cells with rituximab (RTX), the monoclonal anti-CD20 antibody, has been demonstrated as an effective therapy for remission induction and maintenance in severe AAVs.[3,4] In 2011, RTX became the first therapy approved by the Food and Drug Administration for GPA and MPA.

Treatment Principles

As AAV therapies evolve, several fundamental treatment principles continue to guide patient management. First, patients should be stratified by disease severity with treatment tailored to severity of disease. Severe disease, defined as life- or organ-threatening manifestations, includes features, such as rapidly progressive glomerulonephritis, pulmonary hemorrhage, mesenteric ischemia, scleritis, and nervous system involvement and typically requires more aggressive therapy.[41] Limited disease, which encompasses all non–life- or organ-threatening manifestations,

Table 1
Granulomatosis with polyangiitis and microscopic polyangiitis randomized controlled clinical trials

Trial Name	Design	Primary Endpoint	Results
Induction			
CYCLOPS[45]	po-CYC vs IV-CYC in newly diagnosed AAVs with renal involvement	Time to remission	IV-CYC noninferior to po-CYC, lower cumulative dose and less leukopenia with IV, long-term follow-up suggested higher relapse rate with IV
NORAM[39]	MTX vs po-CYC in patients with limited disease	Remission at 6 mo	No difference in remission rates at 6 mo between groups, in long-term follow-up, lower rate of relapse-free survival in MTX group
RAVE[3]	RTX vs po-CYC, new or relapsing AAVs	Steroid-free remission at 6 mo	RTX noninferior to CYC for induction of remission and may be more effective in relapsing disease
RITUXIVAS[4]	IV-CYC + RTX vs IV-CYC + placebo in newly diagnosed AAVs with renal involvement	Remission at 12 mo	RTX + IV-CYC noninferior to IV-CYC alone with similar rates of adverse events
Maintenance			
CYCAZAREM[52]	AZA vs po-CYC in new or relapsing AAVs after induction with po-CYC	Relapse rate	No difference in rates of relapse between the treatment groups
WEGENT[53]	AZA vs MTX after induction with IV-CYC	Adverse events requiring discontinuation of treatment or death	No difference in adverse events and similar relapse rate in both treatment arms, majority of relapses occurred after study medication tapered off
IMPROVE[55]	MMF vs AZA in newly diagnosed AAV patients after induction in CYCLOPS trial	Relapse-free survival	Relapse more common in MMF group with similar rates of adverse events
German Network of Rheumatic Diseases Study[54]	LEF vs MTX in GPA after induction with po-CYC	Relapse rate	Study terminated early because of high incidence of major relapses in MTX arm, although increased frequency of adverse events in LEF arm (LEF dose 30 mg/d)

(continued on next page)

Trial Name	Design	Primary Endpoint	Results
Table 1 *(continued)*			
Dutch Co-Trimoxazole Wegener Study[57]	TMP-SMX vs placebo, in GPA patients during/after remission induction with po-CYC	Disease-free interval	Fewer relapses in patients receiving TMP-SMX, although 20% patients discontinued TMP-SMX due to side effects
WGET[40]	Etanercept vs placebo in addition to CYC (severe) or MTX (limited) for active GPA	Sustained remission for ≥6 mo	Etanercept not effective for remission maintenance, 6 malignancies in etanercept group (all in patients on prior CYC)

including mild renal or pulmonary disease, may not require as potent immunosuppression as severe disease. Similarly, disease flares or relapses should be characterized as limited or severe based on organ systems involved, and this distinction must be taken into account when choosing therapy.

The treatment paradigm is conceptualized in 2 components, namely induction of remission followed by institution of maintenance therapy. This principle arose from recognition of CYC toxicity and desire to minimize and/or avoid CYC exposure if possible. Corticosteroids remain part of all induction regimens in active or relapsing disease and are usually tapered once remission is attained. Some patients are maintained on low-dose corticosteroids during the maintenance period, although at most centers, the aim is for complete discontinuation after remission induction. The optimal tapering regimen and duration of glucocorticoid treatment is not established.

Once remission is induced, structured clinical assessments with urinalysis and basic laboratory tests should be performed regularly to monitor for new organ involvement, treatment response, and drug toxicity.[30] Relapse is common in AAVs, especially after discontinuation of immunosuppression. The optimal duration of maintenance therapy is unknown. Approaching 55% in some studies, relapse rates are highest in the first few years after diagnosis; thus, maintenance immunosuppression is generally continued for approximately 2 years in most patients.[22] Duration of maintenance therapy should be individualized and balance the individual risk of relapse with treatment morbidity. The main cause of death in the first year of AAV diagnosis is infection, accounting for 48% of deaths compared with 19% of deaths due to active vasculitis, so the risk of immunosuppression is not trivial.[38]

Damage, which can be the sequelae of both previous disease activity and treatment-related toxicity, occurs frequently in AAVs.[42] Treatment should be directed to avoid accrual of permanent damage while ensuring immunosuppressive therapy is aimed only at manifestations of active disease, not those reflecting prior damage. Reliable biomarkers that would allow for distinction of active disease from damage or infection, portend relapse, or predict treatment response are lacking in AAVs.[43] Ideally, therapy should be individualized based on a patient's history, comorbidities, disease severity, and pattern of organ involvement.

Induction Therapy

Severe disease

As discussed previously, CYC in combination with high-dose corticosteroids was long considered the standard of care for remission induction therapy in severe AAVs. Complete remission is attainable in greater than 75% of patients treated with oral CYC at doses of 2 mg/kg/d (with dose reductions made for older age and renal insufficiency). Treatment-related morbidity, including hemorrhagic cystitis, malignancy, and infertility, occurs in 50% of patients and is related to cumulative dose.[7,44] In an attempt to minimize CYC exposure, use of pulse intravenous CYC (IV-CYC) was investigated in the CYCLOPS (pulse versus daily oral cyclophosphamide for induction of remission in antineutrophil cytoplasmic antibody-associated vasculitis) trial.[45] In this study comparing daily oral CYC to pulse IV-CYC (15 mg/kg every 2–3 weeks) in newly diagnosed AAVs with renal involvement, there was no difference in time to remission or remission rates between the 2 treatment groups. Patients treated with IV-CYC received lower cumulative doses of CYC and had one-third fewer occurrences of leukopenia. Although this initial study was not powered to detect a difference in relapse rates, long-term follow-up of study participants suggested an increased rate of relapse in those treated with IV-CYC.[46] Thus, CYC regimens are similar in their ability to induce remission with possibly higher relapse rates in IV-CYC, which must be balanced with higher rates of leukopenia and potential infection in daily oral regimens. Deciding between CYC route of administration needs to be an individualized decision between the patient and the treating physician.

B lymphocytes are implicated in the pathogenesis of AAVs by giving rising to autoantibody-producing plasma cells, by contributing to local cytokine production, by acting as antigen-presenting cells, and through the T cell costimulatory pathway. Specific targeting of B lymphocytes with RTX has been shown an effective treatment strategy in severe AAVs. Two randomized trials, including patients with both newly diagnosed and relapsing severe AAVs, demonstrated that RTX was noninferior to CYC for remission induction. In the double-blind, double-dummy randomized controlled Rituximab for ANCA-Associated Vasculitis (RAVE) trial, a single course of RTX (375 mg/m^2 weekly for 4 weeks) was compared with CYC followed by azathioprine (AZA) in 197 AAV patients; all patients received high-dose IV corticosteroids at the beginning of the induction regimen. Patients with serum creatinine greater than 4 mg/dL or alveolar hemorrhage requiring mechanical ventilatory support were excluded from RAVE. The primary endpoint of complete remission and tapering of prednisone at 6 months was achieved by 64% of patients receiving RTX compared with 53% of those receiving CYC, meeting the criteria for noninferiority with similar rates of flare and serious adverse events noted in both groups. In the subset of patients with relapsing disease at trial enrollment, RTX seemed superior to CYC in inducing remission.

Published concurrent with RAVE, the Rituximab versus Cyclophosphamide in ANCA-Associated Renal Vasculitis (RITUXIVAS) study was an open-label trial in newly diagnosed AAVs with renal involvement. Patients were randomized 3:1 to receive RTX (375 mg/m^2 weekly for 4 weeks) plus 2 doses of IV-CYC or pulse IV-CYC alone along with background corticosteroids in both groups. At 12 months, 76% of patients in the RTX-CYC group and 82% of the CYC-only treated patients had achieved sustained remission. Like RAVE, RITUXIVAS concluded an RTX-based regimen was noninferior to a standard CYC induction regimen with similar rates of adverse events. With these studies demonstrating efficacy of RTX as induction therapy, there has been increasing use of RTX as initial therapy in AAVs, especially in patients with concerns about infertility or malignancy. Because those with severe renal dysfunction and respiratory failure were excluded from RAVE, and RITUXIVAS used RTX in combination with CYC, the efficacy of RTX-only regimens in these critically ill patients is not well studied.

Plasma exchange, in conjunction with standard induction therapy, has been used in patients with severe renal disease and/or alveolar hemorrhage. Data suggest plasma exchange may improve renal recovery in those with severe renal disease (creatinine >5.8 mg/dL) or dialysis dependence without any overall mortality benefit.[47] The MEPEX (randomized trial of plasma exchange or high-dosage methylprednisolone as adjunctive therapy for severe renal vasculitis) trial was an open-label study of 1 g pulse methylprednisolone daily for 3 days compared with 7 sessions of plasma exchange for newly diagnosed AAVs with severe renal disease, with all patients getting oral corticosteroids and CYC.[48] At 3 months, 69% of those treated with plasma exchange compared with 49% of those treated with methylprednisolone were alive and dialysis independent. There have been no controlled trials of diffuse alveolar hemorrhage treated with plasma exchange, although retrospective data suggest there may be a benefit.[49] To more definitely answer questions about the role of plasma exchange in AAVs with alveolar hemorrhage and/or severe renal disease, the Plasma Exchange and Glucocorticoids for Treatment of ANCA-Associated Vasculitis (PEXIVAS) is an ongoing randomized, controlled, international study evaluating adjunctive plasma exchange and 2 oral glucocorticoid regimens.[50]

Limited disease

Methotrexate (MTX) can be used to induce remission in limited AAVs as demonstrated in an open-label, randomized trial comparing MTX to CYC.[39] The NORAM (randomized trial of cyclophosphamide versus methotrexate for induction of remission in early systemic antineutrophil cytoplasmic antibody-associated vasculitis) trial randomized patients with newly diagnosed limited AAVs, including patients with mild renal disease, to MTX (15–25 mg weekly) or oral CYC. The primary endpoint of remission at 6 months was achieved in 90% of MTX-treated patients and 94% of CYC-treated patients. Patients receiving MTX took a longer time to achieve remission. At 18 months, higher rates of relapse were seen in those who had been treated with MTX compared with CYC, although a majority of relapses occurred after therapy had been tapered off. The observation of high relapse rates after discontinuation of therapy has led to the standard continuation of maintenance immunosuppression for greater than 12 months in most patients. Follow-up of these patients at a median of 6 years after induction therapy revealed the patients initially treated with MTX had lower rates of relapse-free survival and were treated with immunosuppressive therapy for a longer period of time than those in the CYC group.[51]

Maintenance Therapy

AZA and MTX are the principle conventional immunosuppressive agents used for maintenance remission in AAVs. The CYCAZAREM (A randomized trial of maintenance therapy for vasculitis associated with antineutrophil cytoplasmic autoantibodies) trial randomized 155 patients with newly diagnosed AAVs who had achieved remission on oral CYC to continue treatment with CYC at a lower dose or to switch to AZA.[52] All patients were placed on AZA at 12 months. The primary endpoint of this study was relapse rate at 18 months, which was not significantly different between the 2 treatment groups nor was there a difference in adverse events observed. WEGENT (Azathioprine or methotrexate maintenance for ANCA-associated vasculitis) was a prospective, open-label maintenance trial comparing MTX to AZA in 159 AAV patients, all of whom received IV-CYC for induction.[53] The primary endpoint of this trial was adverse events requiring discontinuation of therapy, with the hypothesis that MTX would better tolerated than AZA. Rates of adverse events and relapse rates were similar between both groups of patients; echoing previous results, a majority of relapses in this trial occurred after discontinuation of maintenance therapy. Thus, MTX and AZA seem comparably efficacious and safe maintenance agents in AAVs. Given renal clearance of MTX, use of MTX in patients with permanent renal damage and reduced creatinine clearance should be avoided, and AZA is likely a safer option in these patients. Similarly, MTX is a known teratogen, making AZA a better option in woman of childbearing potential.

Leflunomide (LEF) is an alternative maintenance agent in AAVs. A trial comparing LEF (30 mg daily) to MTX was terminated early due to a higher incidence of major relapse in the MTX arm, although patients in the LEF arm experienced a significantly higher rate of adverse events.[54] High rates of adverse events and discontinuation of therapy due to intolerability limit the use of LEF as first-line maintenance therapy.

Hypothesizing that mycophenolate mofetil (MMF) would be more effective than AZA in preventing relapse, the IMPROVE (Mycophenolate mofetil versus azathioprine for remission maintenance in antineutrophil cytoplasmic antibody-associated vasculitis) trial randomized 154 newly diagnosed AAV patients to MMF (2000 mg daily) and AZA (2 mg/kg daily) after remission was induced with CYC.[55] At a median follow-up of 36 months, relapse rates were higher in the MMF treatment arm, with a hazard ratio of 1.69 and with no difference in serious adverse events. There have been no head-to-head comparisons of MMF and MTX. Because MMF is less efficacious than AZA in preventing relapse, it is not routinely used as a first-line maintenance therapy in AAVs, although it may have a role in treating patients with refractory disease or those intolerant of other agents.

Bacterial colonization, such as nasal carriage of *Staphylococcus aureus*, has been suggested to play a role in disease induction and relapse in GPA.[56] The role of antistaphylococcal therapy with trimethoprim-sulfamethoxazole (TMP-SMX) was investigated as an adjunctive remission maintenance agent in GPA in a double-blind study of 81 patients, stratified by renal involvement, who were randomized to TMP-SMX (800 mg/160 mg twice daily) or placebo.[57] At 24 months, 82% of TMP-SMX treated patients were in remission compared with 60% of the placebo group with a relative risk of relapse for TMP-SMX of 0.4, although TMP-SMX was discontinued in 20% of patients due to intolerability. The benefit of TMP-SMX seemed most apparent in patients with upper airway disease. Treatment doses of TMP-SMX can be considered an alternative maintenance therapy for GPA patients with mild, localized upper airway disease or an adjunctive therapy in those on other immunosuppressive agents to reduce risk of relapse.

WGET was the first clinical trial in which a biologic was evaluated as a treatment of vasculitis and was based on experimental data suggesting that tumor necrosis factor α (TNF-α) may be an important inflammatory mediator in GPA.[40] WGET randomized 180 GPA patients to received etanercept, an anti–TNF-α agent, or placebo in addition to standard therapy for remission maintenance. Patients with limited disease received MTX as standard therapy and those with severe disease at enrollment were given CYC. There was no difference in rates of sustained remission in those receiving etanercept compared with placebo, and flares were common in both groups. WGET concluded etanercept is not effective for remission maintenance in GPA. Furthermore, 6 patients in the etanercept group developed solid malignancies compared with no malignancies in the placebo group. All of the patients who developed malignancy had received prior CYC; whether TNF blockade had an additive effect on malignancy risk in AAVs is unknown. Given the WGET data, however, anti–TNF-α therapy does not have a routine role in treatment of AAVs.

RTX is an effective maintenance therapy for AAVs. A follow-up of RAVE reported that 48% and 39% of the patients receiving the single course of RTX remained in complete remission at 12 and 18 months, respectively, compared with 39% and 33% of those in the CYC group, again meeting the criteria for noninferiority; RTX again seemed superior in those with relapsing disease with no difference in adverse events between the groups observed.[58] These data suggest that given the prolonged duration of its biologic effects, a single course of RTX has comparable safety and efficacy to continuous conventional immunosuppressive therapy in remission induction and maintenance out to 18 months. Additionally, RTX has proved effectiveness for treatment of severe disease flares regardless of previous treatment history.[59]

The ideal dose and frequency of administration of RTX maintenance remain unknown. An observational study of Mayo Clinic's decade-long experience with repeated RTX treatment of refractory GPA suggests utility in the combination of B-lymphocyte reconstitution and ANCA level in predicting relapse.[60] In this cohort of chronically relapsing patients, all observed relapses occurred after B-cell reconstitution and were temporally accompanied by an increase in PR3 levels (except in 1 patient who was ANCA negative) suggesting that RTX retreatment can be individualized. Other investigators have demonstrated effectiveness of preemptive retreatment approach with RTX.[61,62] A study comparing RTX maintenance at a fixed-dose and interval (1 g every 6 months) to those treated at time of relapse found reduced relapse rates and longer periods of remission in the preemptive retreatment group without an increase in adverse events during the observational period.[61] A trial comparing 2 RTX-based maintenance regimens, 1 based on reconstitution of B lymphocytes and rising ANCAs and the other a strategy of fixed-interval retreatment every 6 months, is ongoing.[63]

There are no controlled studies of RTX expressly for limited disease manifestations. As previously noted, upper airway involvement occurs frequently in GPA and is an independent risk factor for disease relapse. Additionally, persistent, grumbling otolaryngologic disease is common and can lead to accrual of permanent damage, such as nasal bridge collapse, hearing loss, and subglottic stenosis, making treatment of these disease manifestations crucial. The efficacy of RTX for the granulomatous compared with vasculitic manifestations of GPA is debated, with several case series offering conflicting results[64–68] In the largest reported observational cohort looking at RTX solely for otolaryngologic manifestations of GPA, patients given RTX for active ENT disease were greater than 10 times less likely to have active ENT disease compared with patients treated with other therapies[68]; results of this retrospective study suggest RTX may be a useful therapy for granulomatous otolaryngologic disease in GPA.

COMORBIDITY MANAGEMENT

Care of AAV patients must include management of comorbidities known to be associated with AAVs. Thromboembolic events occur with increased frequency in AAVs. First noted in the WGET cohort and subsequently confirmed in other AAV cohorts, patients with AAVs have a rate of thromboembolism that is approximately 20-fold higher than that of the general population and is not associated with antiphospholipid antibodies or other prothrombotic states.[69,70] Clinicians caring for AAV patients need to be aware of this thrombotic risk, which is heightened during periods of disease activity, and screening for deep vein thrombosis or pulmonary embolism may be necessary in the appropriate clinical setting.

Patients with AAVs also demonstrate risk for accelerated atherosclerosis and increased cardiovascular morbidity. AAV patients have increased rates of carotid plaque and aortic stiffness compared with age-matched controls[71] and, more importantly, a 2- to 4-fold increased incidence of myocardial infarction and stroke.[72] Within the first 5 years of AAV diagnosis, approximately 15% of patients experience a cardiovascular event[73]; those with PR3 compared with MPO or negative ANCAs may be at slightly lower risk of cardiovascular morbidity. It is unknown if this cardiovascular risk can be mitigated with early treatment of AAVs because prolonged inflammatory burden may play a role in atherosclerotic disease development. Cardiovascular disease is the major cause of mortality in AAVs after the first year and accounts for one-quarter of all deaths.[38] Management of cardiovascular risk factors, such as hypertension, which occurs in approximately 40% of AAV patients seen in long-term follow-up, and diabetes, occurring in approximately 10% of patients, is critical.[74]

Compared with the general population, patients with AAVs have an increased incidence of malignancy, which is related to the underlying disease and to its therapy. CYC is associated with a dose-related risk of uroepithelial and bladder cancers and hematologic malignancies; however, the threshold dose at which this risk begins is not known. Patients treated with oral CYC have an increased risk of bladder cancer compared with those getting IV-CYC; historical cohorts estimate incidence of bladder cancer in those treated with oral CYC to approach 5% at 10 years.[75] It is not known whether treatment with TNF inhibitors has an additive effect on malignancy in patients previously treated with CYC, as was observed in WGET. With shorter courses of CYC and increased use of pulse IV-CYC, there is decreasing incidence of these malignancies. More recent studies suggest a standardized incidence ratio of cancer in AAVs of 1.6 to 2.0 compared with that of the general population and a possibly higher risk in GPA than in MPA.[76] An analysis of 535 AAV patients found the excess malignancy rate in AAVs was mostly driven by nonmelanoma skin cancers, although bladder cancer, leukemia, and lymphoma were also observed.[77]

FUTURE CONSIDERATIONS

Despite major therapeutic advances in AAVs, there remains a need for therapies that are less toxic, to prevent accrual of treatment-related damage, and those that are effective in maintaining remission and preventing relapse. Future treatment strategies will likely focus on agents targeting elements of the innate and adaptive immune system thought to be involved in AAV pathogenesis. Complement activation, particularly through the alternative pathway, has been implicated in pathogenesis of AAVs, with murine and human studies suggesting the common pathway component C5a plays a key role[78–80]; an inhibitor of C5a is currently being studied in AAVs with renal involvement.[81] B cells and T cells play a role in AAV pathogenesis and disease propagation. Biologic therapies targeting B-cell survival factors and T-cell costimulation are also being studied for AAV maintenance.[82] Improved understanding of molecular mechanisms driving disease as well as increased appreciation of genetic and phenotypic subsets of AAVs should pave the way for more tailored treatment regimens for AAV patients.

EOSINOPHILIC GRANULOMATOSIS WITH POLYANGIITIS
Clinical Features

EGPA commonly presents with asthma/allergic rhinitis, pulmonary infiltrates, and peripheral eosinophilia. Asthma is a cardinal feature of EGPA, and development of asthma and atopy often precede frank vasculitic manifestations by several years. The vasculitic phase of EGPA, which most commonly affects the skin and peripheral nervous system with mononeuritis multiplex occurring in as many as 75% of patients, represents a distinct phase of disease.[83] Both vascular inflammation and eosinophilic infiltration into tissue contribute to the clinical features and organ damage in EGPA.

Antineutrophil Cytoplasmic Antibody

Although the 2012 CHCC classified EGPA as 1 of the AAVs, only approximately half of patients with EGPA are ANCA positive.[84] When present, ANCAs are directed against MPO in 75% of cases. Although significant overlap exists, EGPA may be divided into 2 distinct phenotypes depending on ANCA positivity. ANCA-positive EGPA is more commonly associated with vasculitic manifestations, such as glomerulonephritis, mononeuritis, and pulmonary hemorrhage. ANCA-positive EGPA patients had more upper airway manifestations than the ANCA-negative patients and were at increased risk for relapse, comparable to what is seen in GPA patients with upper airway disease.[85] In contrast, ANCA-negative EGPA was associated with increased risk for cardiac involvement and eosinophilic infiltration of the gastrointestinal tract.

Tissue Biopsy

As in the other AAVs, tissue should be pursued when possible to support a diagnosis of EGPA. Necrotizing small-vessel vasculitis, extravascular granulomas, and eosinophilic infiltration may all be part of the histopathologic spectrum of EGPA; however, this triad of findings rarely coexists in the same biopsy specimen. Demonstration of vasculitis or granuloma may be identical to pathologic findings in MPA or GPA, so consideration of the clinical context is important in differentiating EGPA from the other AAVs. As in the other AAVs, in those with evidence of renal involvement, kidney biopsy is high yield whereas the diagnostic yield of an upper airway biopsy is low. The high frequency of nerve involvement in EGPA makes this an appealing biopsy target; epineural vasculitis with eosinophilia is present in greater than 50% of peripheral nerve biopsies performed.[86]

Treatment

Treatment of EGPA is largely driven by the affected organ-systems and severity of vasculitic disease. The French Vasculitis Study Group has devised a scoring system, the 5-factor score (FFS), to quantify disease activity and severity in EGPA and guide initial management decisions.[87] In the first iteration of the FFS, 1 point was given for presence of each of these 5 factors: cardiac involvement, gastrointestinal ischemia, renal insufficiency, proteinuria, and central nervous system disease (CNS). Patients with greater than 2 of these manifestations are given a score of 2. A more recent version of the FFS included age over 65 and absence of otolaryngologic disease as poor prognostic features, and proteinuria and CNS disease were removed from the score.[88] Because FFS is associated with poor prognosis and mortality, this score in addition to clinical judgment can help guide therapeutic decisions.

Systemic corticosteroids are the mainstay of therapy for EGPA, although the initial dose and tapering schedule are not standardized and are based on individual presentation. In patients with nonsevere disease (FFS 0), corticosteroids alone can often be used. An open-label study of 72 EGPA patients without poor prognostic factors demonstrated that 93% of patients achieved remission on systemic corticosteroids alone; however, one-third of patients relapsed and required additional immunosuppressive agents and 80% of patients required low doses of steroids to maintain remission.[89]

In general, the approach to EGPA treatment parallels the management of GPA and MPA in that initial treatment choice should be tailored to disease severity, pattern of organ involvement, and patient comorbidities, with a step-down approach to less potent immunosuppressives once remission has been induced. CYC in addition to glucocorticoids is recommended for use in patients with severe disease manifestations (FFS 2 or FFS 1 with CNS or cardiac involvement). Some experts also advocate for using CYC as the initial treatment when there is aggressive vasculitic involvement of peripheral nervous system, such as a mononeuritis multiplex. Treatment with CYC substantially reduces mortality in these patients with poor prognostic features.[90] There are no studies of oral CYC versus IV-CYC in EGPA or data on optimal duration of CYC treatment, so practice is usually extrapolated from management of the other AAVs. Similarly, AZA or MTX can be used as induction therapy in place of CYC in patients with mild to moderate disease severity, although there are again few data in EGPA to support this practice. Observational cohorts also support the use of AZA as maintenance therapy or in those with relapsing disease.[91] There are small series of refractory EGPA treated with RTX with improvement in disease activity in both ANCA-positive and ANCA-negative patients, although no controlled data exist.[92]

Promising future therapies for EGPA target pathways involved in disease pathogenesis. A helper T cell type 2 immune response has been implicated in disease pathogenesis with high levels of interleukin (IL)-5 driving the obligatory eosinophilia in EGPA.[93] A monoclonal antibody antagonizing IL-5, mepolizumab, which has been used in hypereosinphilic syndromes, has been investigated in EGPA. Open-label experience with mepolizumab in EGPA suggests safety and a steroid-sparing effect with a larger controlled trial under way.[94,95]

REFERENCES

1. Jennette JC, Falk RJ, Bacon PA, et al. 2012 Revised International Chapel Hill Consensus Conference Nomenclature of Vasculitides. Arthritis Rheum 2013;65: 1–11.
2. Lyons PA, Rayner TF, Trivedi S, et al. Genetically distinct subsets within ANCA-associated vasculitis. N Engl J Med 2012;367:214–23.
3. Stone JH, Merkel PA, Spiera R, et al. Rituximab versus cyclophosphamide for ANCA-associated vasculitis. N Engl J Med 2010;363:221–32.
4. Jones RB, Tervaert JW, Hauser T, et al. Rituximab versus cyclophosphamide in ANCA-associated renal vasculitis. N Engl J Med 2010;363:211–20.
5. Leavitt RY, Fauci AS, Bloch DA, et al. The American College of Rheumatology 1990 criteria for the classification of Wegener's granulomatosis. Arthritis Rheum 1990;33:1101–7.
6. Masi AT, Hunder GG, Lie JT, et al. The American College of Rheumatology 1990 criteria for the classification of Churg-Strauss syndrome (allergic granulomatosis and angiitis). Arthritis Rheum 1990;33:1094–100.
7. Hoffman GS, Kerr GS, Leavitt RY, et al. Wegener's granulomatosis: an analysis of 158 patients. Ann Intern Med 1992;116:488–98.
8. Jennette JC, Falk RJ. Pathogenesis of antineutrophil cytoplasmic autoantibody-mediated disease. Nat Rev Rheumatol 2014;10:463–73.
9. Khan I, Watts RA. Classification of ANCA-associated vasculitis. Curr Rheumatol Rep 2013;15:383.
10. Craven A, Robson J, Ponte C, et al. ACR/EULAR-endorsed study to develop Diagnostic and Classification Criteria for Vasculitis (DCVAS). Clin Exp Nephrol 2013;17:619–21.

11. Xiao H, Heeringa P, Hu P, et al. Antineutrophil cytoplasmic autoantibodies specific for myeloperoxidase cause glomerulonephritis and vasculitis in mice. J Clin Invest 2002;110:955–63.
12. Ohlsson SM, Ohlsson S, Söderberg D, et al. Neutrophils from vasculitis patients exhibit an increased propensity for activation by anti-neutrophil cytoplasmic antibodies. Clin Exp Immunol 2014;176:363–72.
13. Finkielman JD, Lee AS, Hummel AM, et al. ANCA are detectable in nearly all patients with active severe Wegener's granulomatosis. Am J Med 2007;120(7):9–14.
14. Guillevin L, Durand-Gasselin B, Cevallos R, et al. Microscopic polyangiitis: clinical and laboratory findings in eighty-five patients. Arthritis Rheum 1999;42:421–30.
15. Csernok E, Moosig F. Current and emerging techniques for ANCA detection in vasculitis. Nat Rev Rheumatol 2014;10:494–501.
16. Specks U. Controversies in ANCA testing. Cleve Clin J Med 2012;79:S7–11.
17. Weisner O, Russell KA, Lee AS, et al. Antineutrophil cytoplasmic antibodies reacting with human neutrophil elastatse as a diagnostic marker for cocaine-induced midline destructive lesions but not auto-immune vasculitis. Arthritis Rheum 2004;50:2954–65.
18. Kain R, Matsui K, Exner M, et al. A novel class of autoantigens of anti-neutrophil cytoplasmic antibodies in necrotizing and crescentic glomerulonephritis: the lysosomal membrane glycoprotein h-lamp-2 in neutrophil granulocytes and a related membrane protein in glomerular endothelial cells. J Exp Med 1995;181: 585–97.
19. Kain R, Tadema H, McKinney EF, et al. High prevalence of autoantibodies to hLAMP-2 in anti-neutrophil cytoplasmic antibody-associated vasculitis. J Am Soc Nephrol 2012;23:556–66.
20. Roth AJ, Brown MC, Smith RN, et al. Anti-LAMP-2 antibodies are not prevalent in patients with antineutrophil cytoplasmic autoantibody glomerulonephritis. J Am Soc Nephrol 2012;23:545–55.
21. Hogan SL, Nachman PH, Wilkman AS, et al. Prognostic markers in patients with antineutrophil cytoplasmic autoantibody-associated microscopic polyangiitis and glomerulonephritis. J Am Soc Nephrol 1996;7:723–32.
22. Walsh M, Flossmann O, Berden A, et al. Risk factors for relapse of antineutrophil cytoplasmic antibody-associated vasculitis. Arthritis Rheum 2012;64:542–8.
23. Lionaki S, Blyth ER, Hogan SL, et al. Classification of antineutrophil cytoplasmic autoantibody vasculitides. The role of ANCA specificity for myeloperoxidase or proteinase 3 in disease recognition and prognosis. Arthritis Rheum 2012;64:3452–62.
24. Franssen CF, Gans RO, Arends B, et al. Differences between anti-myeloperoxidase- and anti-proteinase 3-associated renal disease. Kidney Int 1995;47:193–9.
25. Mahr A, Katsahian S, Varet H, et al, French Vasculitis Study Group and the European Vasculitis Society. Revisiting the classification of clinical phenotypes of anti-neutrophil cytoplasmic antibody-associated vasculitis: a cluster analysis. Ann Rheum Dis 2013;72:1003–10.
26. Finkielman JD, Merkel PA, Schroeder D, et al, WGET Research Group. Antiproteinase 3 antineutrophil cytoplasmic antibodies and disease activity in Wegener granulomatosis. Ann Intern Med 2007;147:611–9.
27. Birck R, Schmitt WH, Kaelsch IA, et al. Serial ANCA determinations for monitoring disease activity in patients with ANCA-Associated vasculitis: systematic review. Am J Kidney Dis 2006;47:15–23.
28. Tomasson G, Grayson PC, Mahr AD, et al. Value of ANCA measurements during remission to predict a relapse of ANCA-associated vasculitis-a meta-analysis. Rheumatology (Oxford) 2012;51:100–9.

29. Boomsma MM, Stegeman CA, van der Leij MJ, et al. Prediction of relapses in We-gener's granulomatosis by measurement of antineutrophil cytoplasmic antibody levels: a prospective study. Arthritis Rheum 2000;43(9):2025–33.
30. Mukhtyar C, Guillevin L, Cid MC, et al, European Vasculitis Study Group. EULAR recommendations for management of primary small and medium vessel vascu-litis. Ann Rheum Dis 2009;68:310–7.
31. Devaney KO, Travis WD, Hoffman G, et al. Interpretation of head and neck bi-opsies in Wegener's granulomatosis. A pathologic study of 126 biopsies in 70 pa-tients. Am J Surg Pathol 1990;14:555–64.
32. Del Buono EA, Flint A. Diagnostic usefulness of nasal biopsy in Wegener's gran-ulomatosis. Hum Pathol 1991;22:107–10.
33. Borner U, Landis BN, Banz Y, et al. Diagnostic value of biopsies in identifying cytoplasmic antineutrophil cytoplasmic antibody-negative localized Wegener's granulomatosis presenting primarily with sinonasal disease. Am J Rhinol Allergy 2012;26:475–80.
34. Hauer HA, Bajema IM, van Houwelingen HC, et al. Renal histology in ANCA-associated vasculitis: differences between diagnostic and serologic subgroups. Kidney Int 2002;61:80–9.
35. Berden AE, Ferrario F, Hagen EC, et al. Histopathologic classification of ANCA-associated glomerulonephritis. J Am Soc Nephrol 2010;21:1628–36.
36. Ford SL, Polkinghorne KR, Longano A, et al. Histopathologic and clinical predic-tors of kidney outcomes in ANCA-associated vasculitis. Am J Kidney Dis 2014; 63:227–35.
37. Schnabel A, Holl-Ulrich K, Dalhoff K, et al. Efficacy of transbronchial biopsy in pulmonary vaculitides. Eur Respir J 1997;10:2738–43.
38. Flossmann O, Berden A, de Groot K, et al. Long-term patient survival in ANCA-associated vasculitis. Ann Rheum Dis 2011;70:488–94.
39. De Groot K, Rasmussen N, Bacon PA, et al. Randomized trial of cyclophosphamide versus methotrexate for induction of remission in early systemic antineutrophil cyto-plasmic antibody-associated vasculitis. Arthritis Rheum 2005;52:2461–89.
40. Wegener's Granulomatosis Etanercept Research Group. Etanercept plus stan-dard therapy for Wegener's Granulomatosis. N Engl J Med 2005;352:351–61.
41. Stone JH, Wegener's Granulomatosis Etanercept Trial Research Group. Limited versus severe Wegener's granulomatosis: baseline data on patients in the Wege-ner's granulomatosis etanercept trial. Arthritis Rheum 2003;48:2299–309.
42. Seo P, Min YI, Holbrook JT, et al, WGET Research Group. Damage caused by We-gener's granulomatosis and its treatment: prospective data from the Wegener's Granulomatosis Etanercept Trial (WGET). Arthritis Rheum 2005;52:2168–78.
43. Lally L, Spiera RF. Biomarkers in ANCA-associated vasculitis. Curr Rheumatol Rep 2013;15:363–9.
44. Le Guenno G, Mahr A, Pagnoux C, et al. Incidence and predictors of urotoxic adverse events in cyclophosphamide-treated patients with systemic necrotizing vasculitides. Arthritis Rheum 2011;63:1435–45.
45. de Groot K, Harper L, Jayne DR, et al. Pulse versus daily oral cyclophosphamide for induction of remission in antineutrophil cytoplasmic antibody-associated vasculitis: a randomized trial. Ann Intern Med 2009;150:670–80.
46. Harper L, Morgan MD, Walsh M, et al. Pulse versus daily oral cyclophosphamide for induction of remission in ANCA-associated vasculitis: long-term follow-up. Ann Rheum Dis 2012;71:955–60.
47. Pusey CD, Rees AJ, Evans DJ, et al. Plasma exchange in focal necrotizing glomerulonephritis without anti-GBM antibodies. Kidney Int 1991;40:757–63.

48. Jayne DR, Gaskin G, Rasmussen N, et al. Randomized trial of plasma exchange or high-dosage methylprednisolone as adjunctive therapy for severe renal vasculitis. J Am Soc Nephrol 2007;18:2180–8.
49. Klemmer PJ, Chalermskulrat W, Reif MS, et al. Plasmapheresis therapy for diffuse alveolar hemorrhage in patients with small-vessel vasculitis. Am J Kidney Dis 2003;42:1149–52.
50. Walsh M, Merkel PA, Peh CA, et al. Plasma exchange and glucocorticoid dosing in the treatment of anti-neutrophil cytoplasm antibody associated vasculitis (PEXIVAS): protocol for a randomized controlled trial. Trials 2013;14:73.
51. Faurschou M, Westman K, Rasmussen N, et al. Brief Report: long-term outcome of a randomized clinical trial comparing methotrexate to cyclophosphamide for remission induction in early systemic antineutrophil cytoplasmic antibody-associated vasculitis. Arthritis Rheum 2012;34:3472–7.
52. Jayne D, Rasmussen N, Andrassy K, et al. A randomized trial of maintenance therapy for vasculitis associated with antineutrophil cytoplasmic autoantibodies. N Engl J Med 2003;349:36–44.
53. Pagnoux C, Mahr A, Hamidou MA, et al. Azathioprine or methotrexate maintenance for ANCA-associated vasculitis. N Engl J Med 2008;359: 2790–803.
54. Metzler C, Miehle N, Manger K, et al. Elevated relapse rate under oral methotrexate versus leflunomide for maintenance of remission in Wegener's Granulomatosis. Rheumatology (Oxford) 2007;46:1087–91.
55. Hiemstra TF, Walsh M, Mahr A, et al. Mycophenolate mofetil vs azathioprine for remission maintenance in antineutrophil cytoplasmic antibody-associated vasculitis: a randomized controlled trial. JAMA 2010;304:2381–8.
56. Tadema H, Heeringa P, Kallenberg CG. Bacterial infections in Wegener's granulomatosis: mechanisms potentially involved in autoimmune pathogenesis. Curr Opin Rheumatol 2011;23:366–71.
57. Stegeman CA, Tervaert JW, de Jong PE, et al. Trimethoprim-sulfamethoxazole (co-trimoxazole) for the prevention of relapses of Wegener's granulomatosis. Dutch Co-Trimoxazole Wegener Study Group. N Engl J Med 1996;335: 16–20.
58. Specks U, Merkel PA, Seo P, et al. Efficacy of Remission-Induction Regimens for ANCA-Associated Vasculitis. N Engl J Med 2013;369:417–27.
59. Miloslavsky EM, Specks U, Merkel PA, et al. Rituximab for the treatment of relapses in ANCA-associated vasculitis. Arthritis Rheum 2014;43(4):542–57. http://dx.doi.org/10.1002/art.38788.
60. Cartin-Ceba R, Golbin J, Keogh KA, et al. Rituximab for remission induction and maintenance in refractory granulomatosis with polyangiitis (Wegener's): a single-center ten-year experience. Arthritis Rheum 2012;64:3770–8.
61. Smith RM, Jones RB, Guerry M, et al. Rituximab for remission maintenance in relapsing antineutrophil cytoplasmic antibody-associated vasculitis. Arthritis Rheum 2012;64:3760–9.
62. Calich AL, Puéchal X, Pugnet G, et al. Rituximab for induction and maintenance therapy in granulomatosis with polyangiitis (Wegeners). Results of a single-center cohort study on 66 patients. J Autoimmun 2014;50:135–41.
63. Available at: http://clinicaltrials.gov/ct2/show/record/NCT01731561. Accessed August 9, 2014.
64. Holle J, Dubrau C, Herlyn K, et al. Rituximab for refractory granulomatosis with polyangiitis: comparison of efficacy in granulomatous versus vasculitic manifestation. Ann Rheum Dis 2012;71:327–33.

65. Aries PM, Hellmich B, Voswinkel JK, et al. Lack of efficacy of rituximab in Wegener's granulomatosis with refractory granulomatous manifestations. Ann Rheum Dis 2006;65:853–85.
66. Seo P, Specks U, Keogh KA. Efficacy of rituximab in limited Wegener's with refractory granulomatous manifestations. J Rheumatol 2008;35:2017–23.
67. Martinez DP, Chaudhry A, Jones RB, et al. B-cell depletion with rituximab for refractory head and neck Wegener's granulomatosis: a cohort study. Clin Otolaryngol 2009;34:328–35.
68. Lally L, Lebovic R, Huang WT, et al. Effectiveness of rituximab for the otolaryngologic manifestations of granulomatosis with polyangiitis. Arthritis Care Res 2014; 66:1403–9. http://dx.doi.org/10.1002/acr.22311.
69. Merkel PA, Lo GH, Holbrook JT, et al. Brief Communication: high incidence of venous thromboembolic events among patients with Wegener's granulomatosis: the Wegener's Clinical Occurrence of Thrombosis (WeCLOT) Study. Ann Intern Med 2005;142:620–6.
70. Weidner S, Hafezi-Rachti S, Rupprecht HD. Thromboembolic events as a complication of antineutrophil cytoplasmic antibody-associated vasculitis. Arthritis Rheum 2006;55:146–9.
71. de Leeuw K, Sanders JS, Stegeman C, et al. Accelerated atherosclerosis in patients with Wegener's granulomatosis. Ann Rheum Dis 2005;64:753–9.
72. Faurschou M, Mellemkjaer L, Sorensen IJ, et al. Increased morbidity from ischemic heart disease in patients with Wegener's granulomatosis. Arthritis Rheum 2009;60:1187–92.
73. Suppiah R, Judge A, Batra R, et al. A model to predict cardiovascular events in patients with newly diagnosed Wegener's granulomatosis and microscopic polyangiitis. Arthritis Care Res (Hoboken) 2011;63:588–96.
74. Robson J, Doll H, Suppiah R, et al. Damage in the anca-associated vasculitides: long-term data from the European Vasculitis Study group (EUVAS) therapeutic trials. Ann Rheum Dis 2013. http://dx.doi.org/10.1136/annrheumdis-2013-203927.
75. Faurschou M, Sorensen IJ, Mellemkjaer L, et al. Malignancies in Wegener's granulomatosis: incidence and relation to cyclophosphamide therapy in a cohort of 293 patients. J Rheumatol 2008;35:100–5.
76. Mahr A, Heijl C, Le Guenno G, et al. ANCA-associated vasculitis and malignancy: current evidence for cause and consequence relationships. Best Pract Res Clin Rheumatol 2013;27:45–56.
77. Heijl C, Harper L, Flossmann O, et al. Incidence of malignancy in patients treated for antineutrophil cytoplasm antibody-associated vasculitis: follow-up data from European Vasculitis Study Group clinical trials. Ann Rheum Dis 2011;70:1415–21.
78. Xiao H, Schreiber A, Heeringa P, et al. Alternative complement pathway in the pathogenesis of disease mediated by anti-neutrophil cytoplasmic autoantibodies. Am J Pathol 2007;170:52–64.
79. Schreiber A, Xiao H, Jeannette JC, et al. C5a receptor mediates neutrophil activation and ANCA-induced glomerulonephritis. J Am Soc Nephrol 2009;20:289–98.
80. Xiao H, Dairaghi DJ, Powers JP, et al. C5a receptor (CD88) blockade protects against MPO-ANCA GN. J Am Soc Nephrol 2014;25:225–31.
81. Available at: http://clinicaltrials.gov/ct2/show/NCT01363388. Accessed August 9, 2014.
82. Langford CA, Monach PA, Specks U, et al. An open-label trial of abatacept (CTLA4-IG) in non-severe relapsing granulomatosis with polyangiitis (Wegener's). Ann Rheum Dis 2013;73:1376–9.

83. Comarmond C, Pagnoux C, Khellaf M, et al. Eosinophilic granulomatosis with polyangiitis (Churg-Strauss): clinical characteristics and long-term followup of the 383 patients enrolled in the French Vasculitis Study Group cohort. Arthritis Rheum 2013;65:270–81.
84. Sablé-Fourtassou R, Cohen P, Mahr A, et al. Antineutrophil cytoplasmic antibodies in the Churg-Strauss syndrome. Ann Intern Med 2005;143:632–8.
85. Mahr A, Moosig F, Neumann T, et al. Eosinophilic granulomatosis with polyangiitis (Churg-Strauss): evolutions in classification, etiopathogenesis, assessment and management. Curr Opin Rheumatol 2014;26:16–23.
86. Hattori N, Ichimura M, Nagamatsu M, et al. Clinicopathological features of Churg-Strauss syndrome-associated neuropathy. Brain 1999;122:427–39.
87. Guillevin L, Lhote F, Gayraud M, et al. Prognositic factors in polyarteritis nodosa and Churg-Strauss syndrome. A prospective study in 342 patients. Medicine (Baltimore) 1996;75:17–28.
88. Guillevin L, Pagnoux C, Seror R, et al. The Five-Factor Score revisited: assessment of prognoses of systemic necrotizing vasculitides based on the French Vasculitis Study Group (FVSG) cohort. Medicine (Baltimore) 2011;90:19–27.
89. Ribi C, Cohen P, Pagnoux C, et al. Treatment of Churg-Strauss syndrome without poor-prognosis factors: a multicenter, prospective, randomized, open-label study of seventy-two patients. Arthritis Rheum 2008;58:586–94.
90. Gayraud M, Guillevin L, le Toumelin P, et al. Long-term followup of polyarteritis nodosa, microscopic polyangiitis, and Churg-Strauss syndrome: analysis of four prospective trials including 278 patients. Arthritis Rheum 2001;44:666–75.
91. Moosig F, Bremer JP, Hellmich B, et al. A vasculitis centre based management strategy leads to improved outcome in eosinophilic granulomatosis and polyangiitis (Churg-Strauss, EGPA): monocentric experiences in 150 patients. Ann Rheum Dis 2013;72:1011–7.
92. Thiel J, Hässler F, Salzer U, et al. Rituximab in the treatment of refractory or relapsing eosinophilic granulomatosis with polyangiitis (Churg-Strauss syndrome). Arthritis Res Ther 2013;15:133–42.
93. Jakiela B, Szczeklik W, Plutecka H, et al. Increased production of IL-5 and dominant Th2-type response in airways of Churg-Strauss syndrome patients. Rheumatology (Oxford) 2012;51:1887–93.
94. Kim S, Marigowda G, Oren E, et al. Mepolizumab as a steroid-sparing treatment option in patients with Churg-Strauss syndrome. J Allergy Clin Immunol 2010; 125:1336–43.
95. Moosig F, Gross WL, Hermann K, et al. Targeting interleukin-5 in refractory and relapsing Churg-Strauss syndrome. Ann Intern Med 2011;155:341–3.

Small Vessel Vasculitis of the Skin

Robert G. Micheletti, MD[a],*, Victoria P. Werth, MD[a,b]

KEYWORDS

- Small vessel vasculitis of the skin • Cutaneous vasculitis
- Leukocytoclastic vasculitis • Hypersensitivity vasculitis • IgA vasculitis
- Henoch-Schonlein purpura

KEY POINTS

- Small vessel vasculitis of the skin most often presents with palpable purpura.
- Biopsies for routine processing and direct immunofluorescence are important to confirm the diagnosis and identify patients at higher risk of systemic complications.
- A thorough history, examination, and review of systems is important to identify triggers and screen for systemic vasculitis and underlying associated medical conditions.
- The severity of cutaneous involvement, the presence of systemic disease, and the duration of symptoms dictate management.
- Overall, the long-term prognosis of small vessel vasculitis of the skin, including immunoglobulin A vasculitis, is favorable, particularly in the absence of systemic disease.

INTRODUCTION

Small vessel vasculitis of the skin, which classically and most commonly presents as palpable purpura on the lower extremities, has been referred to interchangeably using a number of terms, each of which carries a slightly different shade of meaning. These include "cutaneous leukocytoclastic vasculitis," or simply "leukocytoclastic vasculitis," "hypersensitivity vasculitis," "cutaneous leukocytoclastic angiitis," and "cutaneous small vessel vasculitis," the term for skin-limited small vessel vasculitis favored in the recently revised 2012 Chapel Hill Consensus Criteria.

Regardless of the terminology used, it is important to note that the clinical presentation of small vasculitis in the skin must be considered initially a symptom rather than an entity in and of itself. In other words, when diagnosing skin-limited vasculitis, one

Disclosures: None.
[a] Departments of Dermatology and Medicine, Perelman School of Medicine at the University of Pennsylvania, 3400 Spruce Street, Philadelphia, PA 19104, USA; [b] Departments of Dermatology and Medicine, Philadelphia Veterans Affairs Medical Center, Perelman School of Medicine at the University of Pennsylvania, 3400 Spruce Street, Philadelphia, PA 19104, USA
* Corresponding author.
E-mail address: Robert.Micheletti@uphs.upenn.edu

must first rule out potential systemic manifestations (such as joint, kidney, or gastro-intestinal involvement), underlying causes, and disease associations that affect management and prognosis. In addition, patients may start with skin-limited disease and develop systemic manifestations over time, necessitating careful follow-up. One specific subset of small vessel vasculitis of the skin deserves special mention; immunoglobulin (Ig)A vasculitis (otherwise known as Henoch–Schonlein purpura) is an IgA-mediated syndrome characterized by cutaneous, gastrointestinal, joint, and/or kidney involvement. Though the initial presentation of this condition can be indistinguishable from non–IgA-mediated small vessel skin vasculitis, its management and prognosis is different. Overall, however, small vessel vasculitis of the skin is most often acute and self-limited, and its prognosis is favorable, particularly when internal involvement is absent.

EPIDEMIOLOGY

Small vessel vasculitis of the skin affects both sexes equally and patients of all ages. Studies from Spain have reported an annual incidence of 30 cases of hypersensitivity vasculitis per million adults per year. By contrast, IgA vasculitis has an incidence of 14 cases per million adults per year. A recent, population-based study in Minnesota found the incidence of cutaneous leukocytoclastic vasculitis (including IgA vasculitis as well as other types of small vessel vasculitis) to be almost identical, at 45 cases per million. In children, by contrast, IgA vasculitis is much more common than non-IgA small vessel vasculitis of the skin. The presence of an associated underlying systemic vasculitis, connective tissue disease, or malignancy is much more common in adults than in children.[1–3]

PATHOPHYSIOLOGY

Small vessel vasculitis of the skin is mediated by immune complex deposition in affected vessels.[4] Circulating antigens due to medications, infections, connective tissue disease, or neoplasia are bound by antibodies, forming immune complexes that become lodged and trapped within small vessels, whether in the superficial dermis, most frequently in dependent areas, the joints, the gastrointestinal tract, or the glomeruli. These complexes, in turn, activate complement and induce an inflammatory response that leads to vessel destruction and extravasation of red blood cells. In the case of palpable purpura in the skin, this small vessel involvement accounts for the (usually) small size of the lesions; the complement cascade and subsequent inflammation account for the palpability and symptomatology of the lesions (which often burn); and the red blood cell extravasation results in nonblanching purpura (**Fig. 1**).[5]

ETIOLOGY

About half of cases are idiopathic.[6–8] The remainder are most often either drug induced or post infectious. Antibiotics, and β-lactams in particular, are common culprits, but almost any drug or drug additive can cause vasculitis.[9] Among infectious causes, upper respiratory infections (such as β-hemolytic *Streptococcus* group A) and hepatitis C are commonly implicated; however, numerous infectious triggers have been described.[10,11] Determining a specific cause can be difficult, particularly in the hospitalized setting, when many patients have both a history of recent infection and exposure to numerous medications.

Although palpable purpura is most often due to infection or a drug, it is important to remember that small vessel vasculitis can also be due to an underlying connective

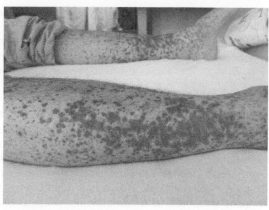

Fig. 1. Typical palpable purpura on the legs of a patient with cutaneous small vessel vasculitis after exposure to an antibiotic.

tissue disease such as systemic lupus erythematosus, Sjögren syndrome, rheumatoid arthritis, or dermatomyositis, and may, in fact, be the presenting sign of such disease. Vasculitis due to underlying connective tissue disease may be associated with more significant internal involvement.[12] Cutaneous manifestations of small vessel vasculitis such as palpable purpura and urticarial lesions can also be a feature of antineutrophil cytoplasmic antibody (ANCA)-associated vasculitis with overlapping involvement of small and medium-sized cutaneous vessels. A small percentage of patients (<5%) may have an underlying hematologic or solid organ malignancy.[13,14] Vasculitis tends to appear 7 to 10 days after exposure to a drug or infectious trigger and a mean of 6 months after the onset of an underlying medical condition. In practice, however, the range and timing of onset varies greatly.[15]

Viral upper respiratory infection or streptococcal pharyngitis frequently precede the onset of IgA vasculitis by 1 to 2 weeks. Overall, about 40% of cases are attributable to an infectious cause, of which very many have been reported.[16] Medication exposure may be to blame in around 20%.[17] In adults, paraneoplastic IgA may be considered; 90% of such patients are male.[18] As with small vessel cutaneous vasculitis as a whole, a significant fraction of cases have no identifiable cause.[19]

Patients with cutaneous vasculitis that is not self-limited or that is refractory or recurrent may be more likely to have an underlying medical illness driving the vasculitis. In such instances, further workup may be required to elucidate the underlying cause. Conversely, recurrence of vasculitis after treatment may herald the relapse of a treated malignancy.

CLINICAL FEATURES
Physical Examination

Small vessel vasculitis in the skin classically presents with crops of purpuric, round, 1- to 3-mm papules that appear over 1 or 2 days on dependent areas, such as the lower legs (see **Fig. 1**). Areas of pressure or trauma, such as the sock lines or underneath sequential compression devices in the hospitalized patient, may be more heavily involved. Although such sites are preferred, lesions can appear anywhere, and for patients confined to bed, clear preference for dependent areas may be less apparent or altered, favoring sites like the back. In IgA vasculitis, palpable purpura above the waist may be a marker for renal vasculitis, but this is controversial.[20,21] The number of lesions may vary from dozens to hundreds. New lesions can appear daily until treatment is initiated or a trigger withdrawn; they resolve over 2 to 3 weeks and slowly fade away, leaving behind postinflammatory hyperpigmentation.[22]

In addition to typical palpable purpura, more subtle, nonpalpable petechial or purpuric lesions may also be present. Larger plaques or even ulcers may develop as purpuric papules coalesce (**Fig. 2**). Vigorous reactions and subsequent ischemic necrosis result in vesicles, pustules, and small hemorrhagic bullae (**Fig. 3**). Hivelike papules and plaques can mimic urticaria but may be the presenting sign of small vessel vasculitis. Unlike true urticaria, these lesions persist longer than 24 hours, burn rather than itch, and leave behind bruiselike, ecchymotic marks on resolution. Some of these patients are best classified as urticarial vasculitis, with either low or normal complement levels.[23]

Absent are manifestations more typical of medium vessel vasculitis, such as subcutaneous nodules, livedo reticularis, retiform purpura, larger hemorrhagic bullae, and more significant ulceration and necrosis. The jagged or retiform shape of purpuric skin fed by medium-sized deep dermal or subcuticular vessels reflects the irregular branching and distribution of downstream small vessels. If such lesions are seen, suspicion for medium vessel vasculitis, namely cutaneous or systemic polyarteritis nodosa, or for ANCA-associated or cryoglobulinemic vasculitis, which can affect both small- and medium-sized cutaneous vessels and present with palpable purpura, should be high.[24]

History

Patients with small vessel vasculitis of the skin may complain of burning, itching, or pain. They may experience aching and uncomfortable swelling of the affected limbs. Or, they may be completely asymptomatic.

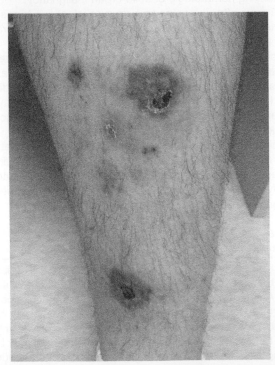

Fig. 2. Coalescing necrotic purpuric plaques with ulceration in a patient with small vessel vasculitis due to underlying hematologic malignancy (chronic lymphocytic leukemia).

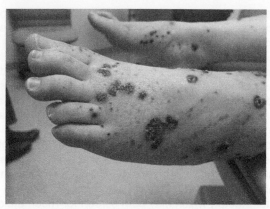

Fig. 3. Hemorrhagic, necrotic bullae in an adult patient with immunoglobulin A vasculitis.

A careful history and review of systems is essential for separating patients with skin-limited vasculitis from those with more significant systemic involvement or an underlying disease. Because such patients may have identical physical findings on initial presentation, the clinical history is of paramount importance. Special attention should be paid to evidence of systemic vasculitis, such as fever, weight loss, and other constitutional symptoms; arthralgias or arthritis; myalgias; abdominal pain, melena, or hematochezia; cough, hemoptysis, or dyspnea; hematuria or frothy urine; sinusitis or rhinitis; and paresthesias, weakness, or foot drop.

In most cases of small vessel vasculitis of the skin, significant systemic manifestations are unlikely. Although arthralgias are fairly common during flares, frank synovitis or arthritis is rare and suggests the presence of systemic disease.[8] If one or more of these symptoms is present, a targeted workup should proceed with the aim of identifying potentially severe extracutaneous manifestations of systemic medium or small vessel vasculitis. In addition to the symptoms discussed, questions about potential triggers, including preceding infectious symptoms, ingestion of prescribed and non-prescribed drugs, and comorbid medical conditions, should be asked.

The hallmark of IgA vasculitis, in addition to typical cutaneous manifestations of small vessel vasculitis, is the presence of gastrointestinal symptoms, such as abdominal pain and gastrointestinal bleeding in 65%, arthralgia or arthritis with periarticular swelling in 63%, and renal involvement with microscopic or gross hematuria in 40%.[17] Because infectious triggers are common, the history should include information about infections, particularly upper respiratory infections, in the preceding weeks, as well as a detailed medical history and medication administration record. Factors that seem to predict renal involvement with IgA vasculitis include age older than 6 years, persistent purpura, severe abdominal pain, and renal symptoms at the time of onset.[25]

INITIAL WORKUP
Laboratory Studies

After a thorough history, review of systems, and physical examination, a systematic and targeted laboratory workup should proceed. No standard protocol for this workup exists, but screening tests should aim to elucidate the underlying cause and extent of organ involvement and should be guided by clinical signs and symptoms. When the presentation is straightforward, there is a recent drug or infectious trigger, and the review of systems is negative, nothing more than a complete blood count, basic metabolic panel, and urinalysis (with micro) may be required. Of these tests, the urinalysis is most essential, because the presence of glomerulonephritis is most likely to change management.

Fecal occult blood testing should be considered in all patients and certainly should be performed if the patient has abdominal symptoms or gastrointestinal bleeding. A chest x-ray should be ordered if the patient complains of dyspnea, and other organ-specific targeted workup should proceed, if warranted, based on review of systems and physical examination.

For those without an obvious cause of vasculitis, a reasonable initial workup includes a complete blood count; basic metabolic panel; urinalysis; liver function tests; infectious serologies, including hepatitis B and C, human immunodeficiency virus, and antistreptolysin-O; and rheumatologic workup, including antinuclear antibody and rheumatoid factor, which may both screen for rheumatoid arthritis and be a surrogate for the presence of mixed cryoglobulins. Second-level tests might include serum protein electrophoresis with immunofixation to look for evidence of a paraprotein; serum C3 and C4 complement levels, which may be low in the context of urticarial vasculitis or systemic lupus and suggest more significant systemic involvement; ANCAs, which are strongly suggestive of ANCA-associated vasculitis, if positive; and cryoglobulins.

Hypersensitivity vasculitis is relatively less common in children compared with adults, whereas IgA vasculitis is much more common. To this end, a more limited initial workup is likely appropriate in children to go along with the history and examination, including complete blood count, basic metabolic panel, urinalysis, fecal occult blood test, and antistreptolysin-O titer. Conversely, given the concern for systemic involvement with IgA vasculitis, special attention should be given to these studies. If an underlying systemic disease is, instead, suspected, then the relevant workup should proceed. The most commonly abnormal laboratory value in small vessel vasculitis of the skin is an elevated erythrocyte sedimentation rate.

Histologic Findings

A skin biopsy should be performed whenever possible to confirm the diagnosis and guide further management; even the most astute clinician can be fooled by conditions that mimic small vessel vasculitis.

DIFFERENTIAL DIAGNOSIS

- Cryoglobulinemic vasculitis
- ANCA-associated vasculitis
- Arthropod bites
- Macular purpura owing to trauma, skin fragility, or anticoagulation
- Platelet dysfunction or deficiency
- Pigmented purpuric dermatosis
- Cholesterol emboli
- Septic emboli
- Livedoid vasculopathy

The type of biopsy performed is dictated by the morphology of the lesion. For manifestations of small vessel vasculitis, a punch biopsy should be sufficient to sample the entire dermis. Because of the natural dynamic progression from immune complex deposition to inflammatory infiltration, vessel disruption, thrombosis, necrosis, and healing, the timing and location of the biopsy are critical. A biopsy performed too early or late may be nondiagnostic. Ideally, a representative lesion should be sampled when it is relatively "fresh" yet well-established, that is, roughly 24 to 48 hours old. Every effort should be made to perform a biopsy the same day the patient is seen, if there are new lesions. If "deeper" lesions, such as subcutaneous nodules or retiform purpura, are present, an appropriately deep punch or wedge biopsy should be performed to sample medium-sized vessels and rule out the presence of a medium or small-to-medium vessel vasculitis.

The prototypical findings of leukocytoclastic vasculitis include a neutrophilic infiltrate of superficial and mid dermal small blood vessels, granulocytic debris and nuclear dust (leukocytoclasis), fibrinoid necrosis and disruption of vessel walls, and extravasation of red blood cells into the surrounding tissue (**Fig. 4**).[5] A mixed inflammatory infiltrate may also be present, particularly in older lesions. The presence of tissue eosinophilia suggests the vasculitis may be drug-induced.[26] Some have suggested that the severity of the histologic changes and the depth of the inflammatory infiltrate may predict disease severity and systemic involvement or even the presence of underlying malignancy.[27] The presence of granulomatous vasculitis is suggestive of granulomatosis with polyangiitis or eosinophilic granulomatosis with polyangiitis.

It is important to note that these histologic patterns can be seen in any vasculitic syndrome and are not specific for any particular entity. Infections, insect bite reactions, neutrophilic dermatoses (Sweet syndrome, pyoderma gangrenosum), and ulcers due to other causes may all exhibit leukocytoclastic vasculitis secondary to the primary process. Clinical–pathologic correlation, as always, is necessary before settling on a final diagnosis.

Whenever possible, a second biopsy should be performed for direct immunofluorescence studies.[28] Detection of immune complex deposition may have prognostic significance. The presence of IgA deposits in vessel walls is the defining pathologic feature of IgA vasculitis[29] and increases the likelihood of the renal, joint, and gastrointestinal symptoms seen in that syndrome. Meanwhile, the presence of IgM in lesional skin may correlate with renal involvement[30] or cryoglobulinemia.[31] A continuous band of C3 or IgG at the dermoepidermal junction (positive lupus band test) may suggest hypocomplementemic urticarial vasculitis and underlying systemic lupus erythematosus.

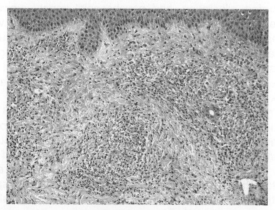

Fig. 4. Infiltration of superficial and mid dermal small blood vessels with neutrophils, leukocytoclasis, fibrinoid necrosis and disruption of vessel walls, and extravasation of red blood cells. Stained with hematoxylin—eosin stain, original magnification ×100.

Proper selection of the biopsy site is again critical, because immune complexes are most likely to be seen in early lesions between 8 and 24 hours of age. Because the subsequent inflammatory cascade destroys the immune complexes, older lesions may be falsely negative. Biopsies for direct immunofluorescence should be taken from lesional skin, and the specimen should be placed in Michel's medium or normal saline for processing.

Finally, the term "leukocytoclastic vasculitis" is sometimes used improperly on histology reports to describe isolated perivascular infiltrates that lack vessel wall infiltration or fibrinoid necrosis. Although such specimens may, in truth, represent early small vessel vasculitis, they are not diagnostic of the disease and may lead to confusion. It is therefore important to read the pathology report in detail, including direct immunofluorescence study, if done, and not rely solely on the printed line diagnosis.

Initial Management

Once a diagnosis of small vessel vasculitis in the skin has been made, the most important initial step in management is, as outlined, evaluation for possible systemic involvement, followed by workup for underlying conditions, as dictated by the examination, history, and review of systems. Initial therapy is dictated by the results of these investigations, because more aggressive systemic therapy is necessary in the case of renal or other organ involvement, and cessation of a causative agent or treatment of an underlying condition is indicated, if one is identified.

Once systemic involvement has been excluded, the treatment of cutaneous small vessel vasculitis should be focused on symptom management. Because the majority of cases affect only the skin, are acute, and self-limited, aggressive immunosuppressive therapy is generally not advisable. Identifiable triggers should be eliminated or treated. Prolonged standing should be avoided. Rest and elevation and use of compression stockings can be helpful to decrease stasis-related immune complex deposition and accelerate healing of ulcers on the lower legs. Topical steroids can relieve itch or burning but do not prevent new lesions. More than half of patients require no systemic treatment.[6]

Subsequent Management

Systemic therapies are indicated for severe, intractable, or recurrent disease. The associated discomfort, ulceration, and psychosocial impact warrant intervention. Any initial episode that is not self-limited and lasts longer than a few weeks likely warrants systemic treatment, even if it is relatively asymptomatic. Unfortunately, there is a dearth of high-quality data to direct management, and more than 1 agent is often tried before success is achieved. For patients with chronic small vessel vasculitis of the skin, complete resolution or cure may remain elusive, but often anti-inflammatory medications work without the need for systemic glucocorticoids.

Initial, long-term treatment options include colchicine (0.6 mg 2–3 times per day, if tolerated). This medication has been reported useful for skin and joint symptoms in open label studies, inducing prompt resolution of cutaneous vasculitis. Although it did not show significant benefit in a randomized, controlled trial of 20 patients (the only study of its kind for cutaneous small vessel vasculitis), the enrolled patients were refractory to other therapies and a subset of them did respond and flared when taken off the medication.[32] Dosing may be limited by gastrointestinal side effects.

The use of dapsone (50–200 mg/d), which has antineutrophilic effects, is supported by anecdotal experience and small case series.[33] It is contraindicated in patients with glucose-6-phosphate dehydrogenase deficiency, and it can cause methemoglobinemia and anemia due to hemolysis, necessitating regular laboratory monitoring. It may be combined with colchicine when response to monotherapy with either medication is incomplete. Other options include hydroxychloroquine (200–400 mg/d),[34] which is helpful primarily in urticarial vasculitis; pentoxifylline (400–1200 mg/d),[35] which can also be combined with dapsone; and nonsteroidal anti-inflammatory agents like indomethacin, which may help to alleviate symptoms. The use of these agents is supported only by case series and anecdotal data.

Systemic corticosteroids, with initial doses of 0.5 to 1 mg/kg per day of prednisone, are recommended for those with severe, necrotic lesions or serious systemic manifestations, such as renal or gastrointestinal involvement. The response to such therapy is usually rapid, and the dose should be tapered slowly to prevent rebound. Long-term therapy may not be required if the process is self-limited. Unfortunately, in cases of chronic cutaneous vasculitis, systemic steroids, with their associated side effects, are not a good long-term option. In a Cochrane review of randomized controlled trials, early treatment with corticosteroids at the time of diagnosis showed no benefit for preventing renal complications of IgA vasculitis.[36] Because corticosteroids do not seem to prevent renal complications of IgA vasculitis, their prophylactic use is not recommended. However, they do ameliorate joint and abdominal pain and seem to accelerate the resolution of renal symptoms.[25] In patients with severe extrarenal symptoms and in those who develop renal disease, their use should be considered.

When none of these agents is effective or tolerated, or if the vasculitis is chronic or refractory, immunosuppressive medications such as azathioprine (50–200 mg/d, if thiopurine methyltransferase levels are normal),[37] methotrexate (15–25 mg/wk), with folic acid supplementation,[38] and mycophenolate mofetil (2–3 g/d)[39] can be considered, balancing the risks of these agents against the severity of the skin condition and whatever systemic manifestations are present. Stronger and more toxic agents such as cyclophosphamide may be effective. The tumor necrosis factor inhibitors, especially infliximab, may be effective for small vessel vasculitis of the skin but can also cause vasculitis.[40] Rituximab has been used in some refractory cases.[41]

Prognosis

Most episodes of small vessel vasculitis of the skin are self-limited, resolve over 3 to 4 weeks with residual hyperpigmentation, and do not recur. In general, systemic involvement (if found) is minimal. However, serious internal organ dysfunction does rarely occur. Prognosis depends on the severity of organ involvement as well as any underlying associated medical disorder. A certain number of patients, perhaps 8% to 10%, develop chronic or recurrent vasculitis.[8] Despite this, most cases have an overall good prognosis.[6]

The usual duration of IgA vasculitis is between several weeks to a few months (average of 4 weeks).[42] No therapy has been proven to shorten the duration of disease. Up to one third of patients have persistent or recurrent disease for as long as 6 months. Close follow-up, with frequent repeat urinalysis and blood pressure monitoring, should be continued for at least that long.[43] The prognosis of IgA vasculitis is generally favorable but depends mostly on the severity of renal disease. Even children with gross hematuria usually do well. However, progressive glomerular disease and renal failure may occur in 1% to 3%, so patients with hematuria or proteinuria should be carefully followed for late deterioration of renal function.[42] Renal insufficiency and long-term sequelae are more common in adults. Still, persistent, usually mild nephropathy occurs in only 8% of adult patients.[17]

SUMMARY

Despite the generally good prognosis of small vessel vasculitis of the skin, this group of conditions can be a considerable source of morbidity, especially for those afflicted with systemic or chronic/recurrent disease. The dearth of high-quality data to guide the diagnosis, management, and follow-up of cutaneous vasculitis is an ongoing area of need. Larger series with substantial follow-up and well-designed and controlled therapeutic trials are needed to help to develop evidence-based guidelines for the evaluation and treatment of these conditions.

REFERENCES

1. García-Porrúa C, González-Gay MA. Comparative clinical and epidemiological study of hypersensitivity vasculitis versus Henoch-Schönlein purpura in adults. Semin Arthritis Rheum 1999;28(6):404–12.
2. Blanco R, Martínez-Taboada VM, Rodríguez-Valverde V, et al. Cutaneous vasculitis in children and adults. Associated diseases and etiologic factors in 303 patients. Medicine (Baltimore) 1998;77(6):403–18.
3. Arora A, Wetter DA, Gonzalez-Santiago TM, et al. Incidence of leukocytoclastic vasculitis, 1996 to 2010: a population-based study in Olmsted County, Minnesota. Mayo Clin Proc 2014. [Epub ahead of print].
4. Mackel SE, Jordon RE. Leukocytoclastic vasculitis. A cutaneous expression of immune complex disease. Arch Dermatol 1982;118(5):296–301.
5. Carlson JA. The histological assessment of cutaneous vasculitis. Histopathology 2010;56(1):3.
6. Martinez-Taboada VM, Blanco R, Garcia-Fuentes M. Clinical features and outcome of 95 patients with hypersensitivity vasculitis. Am J Med 1997;102: 186–91.
7. Gyselbrecht L, De Keyser F, Ongenae K. Etiological factors and underlying conditions in patients with leukocytoclastic vasculitis. Clin Exp Rheumatol 1996; 14:665–8.
8. Russell JP, Gibson LE. Primary cutaneous small vessel vasculitis: approach to diagnosis and treatment. Int J Dermatol 2006;45(1):3–13.
9. Lowry MD, Hudson CF, Callen JP. Leukocytoclastic vasculitis caused by drug additives. J Am Acad Dermatol 1994;30(5 Pt 2):854–5.
10. Greco F, Sorge A, Salvo V, et al. Cutaneous vasculitis associated with Mycoplasma pneumoniae infection: case report and literature review. Clin Pediatr (Phila) 2007;46:451.
11. Kim HM, Park YB, Maeng HY, et al. Cutaneous leukocytoclastic vasculitis with cervical tuberculous lymphadenitis: a case report and literature review. Rheumatol Int 2006;26:1154.
12. Barile-Fabris L, Hernandez-Cabrera MF, Barragan-Garfias JA. Vasculitis in systemic lupus erythematosus. Curr Rheumatol Rep 2014;16(9):440.
13. Loricera J, Calvo-Rio V, Ortiz-Sanjuan F, et al. The spectrum of paraneoplastic cutaneous vasculitis in a defined population: incidence and clinical features. Medicine (Baltimore) 2013;92(6):331–43.
14. Podjasek JO, Wetter DA, Pittelkow MR, et al. Cutaneous small-vessel vasculitis associated with solid organ malignancies: the Mayo Clinic experience, 1996 to 2009. J Am Acad Dermatol 2012;66(2):e55–65.
15. Carlson JA, Cavaliere LF, Grant-Kels JM. Cutaneous vasculitis: diagnosis and management. Clin Dermatol 2006;24(5):414–29.

16. Rigante D, Castellazzi L, Bosco A, et al. Is there a crossroad between infections, genetics, and Henoch-Schönlein purpura? Autoimmun Rev 2013;12(10): 1016–21.
17. Calvo-Río V, Loricera J, Mata C, et al. Henoch-Schönlein purpura in northern Spain: clinical spectrum of the disease in 417 patients from a single center. Medicine (Baltimore) 2014;93(2):106–13.
18. Zurada JM, Ward KM, Grossman ME. Henoch-Schönlein purpura associated with malignancy in adults. J Am Acad Dermatol 2006;55(Suppl 5):S65–70.
19. Coppo R, Amore A, Gianoglio B. Clinical features of Henoch-Schönlein purpura. Italian Group of Renal Immunopathology. Ann Med Interne (Paris) 1999;150(2): 143–50.
20. Tancrede-Bohin E, Ochonisky S, Vignon-Pennamen MD, et al. Schonlein-Henoch purpura in adult patients. Predictive factors for IgA glomerulonephritis in a retrospective study of 57 cases. Arch Dermatol 1997;133(4):438–42.
21. Poterucha TJ, Wetter DA, Gibson LE, et al. Correlates of systemic disease in adult Henoch-Schönlein purpura: a retrospective study of direct immunofluorescence and skin lesion distribution in 87 patients at Mayo Clinic. J Am Acad Dermatol 2012;67(4):612–6.
22. Fiorentino DF. Cutaneous vasculitis. J Am Acad Dermatol 2003;48(3):311–40.
23. Loricera J, Calvo-Rio V, Mata C, et al. Urticarial vasculitis in northern Spain: clinical study of 21 cases. Medicine (Baltimore) 2014;93(1):53–60.
24. Xu LY, Esparza EM, Anadkat MJ, et al. Cutaneous manifestations of vasculitis. Semin Arthritis Rheum 2009;38(5):348–60.
25. Ronkainen J, Koskimies O, Ala-Houhala M, et al. Early prednisone therapy in Henoch-Schönlein purpura: a randomized, double-blind, placebo-controlled trial. J Pediatr 2006;149(2):241–7.
26. Bahrami S, Malone JC, Webb KG, et al. Tissue eosinophilia as an indicator of drug-induced cutaneous small-vessel vasculitis. Arch Dermatol 2006;142:155.
27. Podjasek JO, Wetter DA, Wieland CN, et al. Histopathologic Findings in Cutaneous Small-Vessel Vasculitis Associated With Solid-Organ Malignancy. Br J Dermatol 2014. [Epub ahead of print].
28. Minz RW, Chhabra S, Singh S, et al. Direct immunofluorescence of skin biopsy: perspective of an immunopathologist. Indian J Dermatol Venereol Leprol 2010; 76:150.
29. Jennette JC, Falk RJ, Bacon PA, et al. 2012 revised International Chapel Hill Consensus Conference Nomenclature of Vasculitides. Arthritis Rheum 2013; 65(1):1–11.
30. Takeuchi S, Soma Y, Kawakami T. IgM in lesional skin of adults with Henoch-Schönlein purpura is an indication of renal involvement. J Am Acad Dermatol 2010;63(6):1026–9.
31. Gibson LE. Cutaneous vasculitis update. Dermatol Clin 2001;19:603–15.
32. Sais G, Vidaller A, Jucqla A. Colchicine in the treatment of cutaneous leukocytoclastic vasculitis. Results of a prospective, randomized controlled trial. Arch Dermatol 1995;131:1399.
33. Fredenberg MF, Malkinson FD. Sulfone therapy in the treatment of leukocytoclastic vasculitis. Report of three cases. J Am Acad Dermatol 1987;16(4):772–8.
34. Lopez LR, Davis KC, Kohler PF, et al. The hypocomplementemic urticarial-vasculitis syndrome: therapeutic response to hydroxychloroquine. J Allergy Clin Immunol 1984;73:600–3.
35. Nurnberg W, Grabbe J, Czarnetzki BM. Urticarial vasculitis syndrome effectively treated with dapsone and pentoxifylline. Acta Derm Venereol 1995;75:54–6.

36. Chartapisak W, Opastirakul S, Hodson EM, et al. Interventions for preventing and treating kidney disease in Henoch-Schonlein purpura (HSP). Cochrane Database Syst Rev 2009;(3):CD005128.
37. Callen JP, Spencer LV, Burruss JB, et al. An effective, corticosteroid-sparing therapy for patients with recalcitrant cutaneous lupus erythematosus or with recalcitrant cutaneous leukocytoclastic vasculitis. Arch Dermatol 1991;127: 515–22.
38. Jorizzo JL, White WL, Wise CM, et al. Low dose weekly methotrexate for unusual neutrophilic vascular reactions: cutaneous polyarteritis nodosa and Behcet's disease. J Am Acad Dermatol 1991;24:973–8.
39. Haeberle MT, Adams WB, Callen JP. Treatment of severe cutaneous small-vessel vasculitis with mycophenolate mofetil. Arch Dermatol 2012;148(8):887–8.
40. Mang R, Ruzicka T, Stege H. Therapy for severe necrotizing vasculitis with infliximab. J Am Acad Dermatol 2004;51:321.
41. Chung L, Funke AA, Chakravarty EF, et al. Successful use of rituximab for cutaneous vasculitis. Arch Dermatol 2006;142(11):1407–10.
42. Saulsbury FT. Clinical update: Henoch-Schönlein purpura. Lancet 2007; 369(9566):976–8.
43. Jauhola O, Ronkainen J, Koskimies O, et al. Renal manifestations of Henoch-Schonlein purpura in a 6-month prospective study of 223 children. Arch Dis Child 2010;95(11):877–82.

Polyarteritis Nodosa

Lindsy Forbess, MD, MSc[a],*, Serguei Bannykh, MD, PhD[b]

KEYWORDS

- Polyarteritis nodosa • Vasculitis • Systemic necrotizing vasculitis
- Medium vessel vasculitis

KEY POINTS

- Polyarteritis nodosa (PAN) is a necrotizing systemic medium vessel vasculitis, which is typically antineutrophil cytoplasmic antibody (ANCA) negative and rarely affects the lungs.
- With the decline of hepatitis B virus (HBV) and the evolving definitions of vasculitis, PAN is becoming a rare disease.
- Variants of PAN include single-organ disease and cutaneous PAN. PAN can be idiopathic or secondary to other causes, typically viral infections (HBV, hepatitis C virus, and human immunodeficiency virus).
- Treatment is mostly borrowed from literature involving ANCA–associated vasculitides and consists of corticosteroids, with the addition of immunosuppressive agents if corticosteroids are not tolerated, cannot be tapered, or if prognosis is poor.
- Treatment of viral-associated PAN is aimed at treating the underlying virus, with escalation of immunosuppression in severe cases.

INTRODUCTION

Polyarteritis nodosa (PAN) is a systemic necrotizing vasculitis, which typically affects medium-sized muscular arteries, particularly affecting the visceral, renal, and soft tissue vasculature.[1] PAN can affect virtually every organ but has a striking tendency to spare the lungs.[1] Small arteries may be involved, but small vessels, including arterioles, capillaries, and venules, are usually spared. Therefore, glomerulonephritis and pulmonary capillaritis are not part of the spectrum of PAN.[2] Antineutrophil cytoplasmic antibodies (ANCAs) are typically negative.[2] These characteristics help differentiate PAN from other systemic necrotizing vasculitides.

PAN may be idiopathic or triggered by specific agents. The most typical is hepatitis B virus (HBV), although other viruses such as hepatitis C virus (HCV) and human immunodeficiency virus (HIV) may occasionally be detected.[3] PAN is a systemic disease, but variants are single-organ disease and cutaneous PAN (cPAN).[2,4]

[a] Department of Rheumatology, Cedars-Sinai Medical Center, 8700 Beverly Boulevard, Los Angeles, CA 90048, USA; [b] Department of Pathology, Cedars-Sinai Medical Center, 8700 Beverly Boulevard, Los Angeles, CA 90048, USA
* Corresponding author. 8700 Beverly Boulevard, Suite B131, Los Angeles, CA 90048.
E-mail address: lindsy.forbess@cshs.org

Rheum Dis Clin N Am 41 (2015) 33–46
http://dx.doi.org/10.1016/j.rdc.2014.09.005
0889-857X/15/$ – see front matter

CLASSIFICATION

Since the early description of periarteritis nodosa by Kussmaul and Maier in 1866,[5] investigators have attempted to develop systems for nomenclature and classification of PAN. The American College of Rheumatology (ACR) proposed classification criteria for PAN in 1990, which took into account clinical, laboratory, radiographic, and histologic features of the disease (**Table 1**).[6] Three of 10 criteria showed a sensitivity of 82.2% and specificity of 86.6% for the classification of PAN.[6] As knowledge has progressed, the ACR criteria seem to have important limitations.[7] They do not recognize microscopic polyangiitis (MPA) as a distinct disease entity from PAN and do not take into account ANCA testing.

The formal distinction between PAN and MPA was made at the Chapel Hill Consensus Conference (CHCC) in 1994.[8] The former was limited to necrotizing inflammation of medium-sized and small arteries without involvement of smaller vessels (ie, arterioles, venules, or capillaries), whereas the latter was described as a pauci-immune (few or no immune deposits) necrotizing vasculitis affecting small vessels, with or without involvement of medium-sized arteries. The CHCC proposed pathologic definitions for vasculitis but recognized that histologic data would not be available for all patients.[8] Surrogate markers of vasculitis and the importance of ANCA were introduced, but neither was included in the definitions of vasculitis.

Table 1
1990 ACR criteria for the classification of PAN

Criterion (≥3 Are Necessary)	Definition
Weight loss ≥4 kg	Loss of ≥4 kg of body weight since the illness began, not caused by dieting or other factors
Livedo reticularis	Mottled reticular pattern over the skin in portions of the extremities or torso
Testicular pain or tenderness	Pain or tenderness of the testicles not caused by infection, trauma, or other causes
Myalgias, weakness, or leg tenderness	Diffuse myalgias (excluding shoulder and hip girdle), weakness of muscles, or tenderness of leg muscles
Mononeuropathy or polyneuropathy	Development of mononeuropathy, multiple mononeuropathies, or polyneuropathy
Diastolic BP >90 mm Hg	Development of hypertension with the diastolic BP >90 mm Hg
Increased blood urea nitrogen (BUN) or creatinine level	Increase of BUN >40 mg/dL or creatinine level >1.5 mg/dL, not caused by dehydration or obstruction
HBV	Presence of hepatitis B surface antigen or antibody in serum
Arteriographic abnormality	Arteriogram showing aneurysms or occlusions of the visceral arteries, not caused by arteriosclerosis, fibromuscular dysplasia, or other noninflammatory causes
Biopsy of small or medium-sized artery containing polymorphonuclear neutrophils	Histologic changes showing the presence of granulocytes or granulocytes and mononuclear leukocytes in the artery wall

Data from Lightfoot RW Jr, et al. The American College of Rheumatology 1990 criteria for the classification of polyarteritis nodosa. Arthritis Rheum 1990;33(8):1088–93.

The importance of negativity of ANCA in PAN was subsequently emphasized by the French Vasculitis Study Group (FVSG) and in the updated 2012 Chapel Hill consensus definitions.[9,10]

Both the ACR criteria (1990) and the CHCC definitions (1994) have been criticized, because there is discordance when they are applied to patient cohorts, with the ACR criteria tending to overdiagnose PAN compared with the CHCC definitions.[7,11,12] Although these two criteria have been adopted and used for diagnostic purposes, this was not their intended purpose. The ACR criteria (1990) were designed as classification criteria, to provide a standard method of describing groups of patients for research and to distinguish one type of vasculitis from another, but not to distinguish vasculitis from other diseases. The CHCC criteria aimed to reach a consensus on the names of major vasculitides and provide working definitions of various types of vasculitis but were not intended to be used as diagnostic or classification criteria.

A consensus algorithm was developed by Watts and colleagues[13] by combining ACR and CHCC criteria, ANCA testing, and surrogate markers of vascular inflammation (clinical, laboratory, and imaging tests), for the classification of PAN and ANCA-associated vasculitis (AAV) for use in epidemiologic studies (**Fig. 1**).[14] To enter this stepwise algorithm, patients must have signs or symptoms compatible with PAN or AAV without other conditions being more likely. This algorithm allows patients to be classified into one category, without many unclassified patients or overlapping diagnoses.[13,14] Diagnostic criteria have also been attempted and through a survey of 949 patients in the FVSG, HBV positivity, peripheral neuropathy, arteriographic abnormalities, as well as the absence of ANCA, asthma, ear nose and throat signs, glomerulopathy, and cryoglobulinemia were predictive of PAN diagnosis.[15]

Despite these efforts, criteria for systemic vasculitides, particularly for PAN, still remain unsatisfactory, and there is a large international collaborative effort aimed to establish better diagnostic and classification criteria.[16,17]

EPIDEMIOLOGY/RISK FACTORS

PAN is a rare disease that affects all racial groups, affecting men more often than women, and occurring primarily in patients in their 40s to 60s.[1,18] Children can also be affected by PAN.[19] Most cases of PAN are idiopathic, although HBV, HCV, HIV, parvovirus B19, and hairy cell leukemia have been implicated in the pathogenesis of some cases.[2] In these settings, PAN is termed secondary PAN. HBV-associated and HCV-associated PAN are more prevalent in developed countries, whereas HIV-associated PAN is more prevalent in underdeveloped countries.[20]

PAN is becoming a rare disease. This situation may be caused in part by the decrease in HBV infection as a result of widespread vaccination, as well as other systemic necrotizing vasculitides being increasingly recognized as a result of increased awareness and improved diagnostic techniques.[21] Reports in the 1970s estimated that HBV, the most common and better characterized trigger of PAN, accounted for one-third of the cases of PAN. Since the essential disappearance of contaminated blood transfusions and the large use of vaccinations against people at risk for HBV, the frequency of HBV is less than 5% in developed countries.[21]

Given the confusion of classification and the changing definition of the disease, estimating the true incidence and prevalence of PAN is difficult. Cohorts of patients with PAN before the 1990s almost certainly included patients with a mixture of PAN and MPA, and likely other forms of vasculitis as well. The development of classification criteria and nomenclature for PAN in the 1990s enabled epidemiologic studies to be performed, although with aforementioned limitations.[7,12]

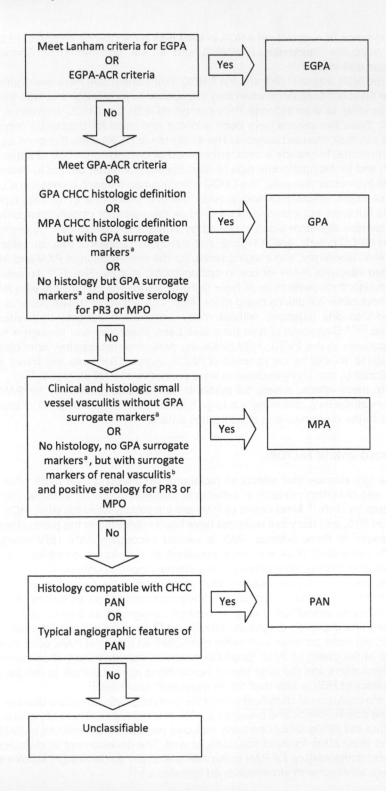

Meet Lanham criteria for EGPA
OR
EGPA-ACR criteria

Yes → EGPA

No ↓

Meet GPA-ACR criteria
OR
GPA CHCC histologic definition
OR
MPA CHCC histologic definition
but with GPA surrogate
markers[a]
OR
No histology but GPA surrogate
markers[a] and positive serology
for PR3 or MPO

Yes → GPA

No ↓

Clinical and histologic small
vessel vasculitis without GPA
surrogate markers[a]
OR
No histology, no GPA surrogate
markers[a], but with surrogate
markers of renal vasculitis[b]
and positive serology for PR3 or
MPO

Yes → MPA

No ↓

Histology compatible with CHCC
PAN
OR
Typical angiographic features of
PAN

Yes → PAN

No ↓

Unclassifiable

Prevalence estimates of PAN are about 31 cases/million.[22,23] The annual incidence ranges from 0 to 8/million in European countries and Australia.[18,24,25] Estimates of the annual incidence of PAN range from 4.6/million in England, 9/million in Olmsted County, Minnesota to 77/million in hepatitis B–endemic Alaskan Eskimo populations.[3] In Germany and Spain, the PAN incidence is low (0.3 and 0.9/million, respectively).[24] There are some regional variations in the incidence of PAN even within the same country, but this may be caused in part by differences in case definitions and ascertainment.[24]

A genetic component of PAN was recently recognized. Families with multiple cases of cPAN and systemic PAN consistent with autosomal recessive inheritance were identified, and exome sequencing of genomic DNA was performed.[26] These patients, who were of Georgian Jewish or German ancestry, as well as unrelated affected patients of Turkish ancestry, were found to have a loss of function mutation of the gene encoding adenosine deaminase 2 (ADA2). ADA2 is both the major extracellular adenosine deaminase and an adenosine deaminase–related growth factor. The clinical presentation of PAN in these patients was variable in terms of age of onset, organ involvement, and severity, even among families, although almost all cases showed disease onset in childhood. This study provides important information about the genetic susceptibility and potential pathophysiology for at least a subset of patients with PAN.[26]

PATHOGENESIS

The pathogenesis of PAN remains poorly understood. In those subsets of cases related to HBV, immune complexes are believed to play a role.[21] However, glomerulonephritis, a characteristic immune complex–mediated lesion, is not associated with PAN. Complement consumption, common in other immune complex–mediated diseases (such as systemic lupus erythematosus), is unusual in PAN. It is postulated that in PAN, viral antigens trigger the complement cascade, resulting in a neutrophil-rich and lymphocyte-rich inflammatory infiltrate within the arterial media, which leads to fibrosis, thrombosis, or aneurysmal degeneration.[1] The mechanism by which immune complexes lead to medium-sized arterial inflammation and yet spare smaller vessels (ie, arterioles, capillaries, and venules) is unknown.

CLINICAL FEATURES

PAN may affect virtually every organ system and has a wide constellation of clinical manifestations (**Table 2**).[27] Constitutional symptoms, such as fever, myalgias, and weight loss, are found in up to 90% of patients with PAN.[27] The peripheral nervous

◄ ───

Fig. 1. Classification algorithm. EGPA, eosinophilic granulomatosis with polyangiitis; GPA, granulomatosis with polyangiitis; MPO, myeloperoxidase; PAN, polyarteritis nodosa; PR3, proteinase-3. [a] GPA surrogate markers refer to symptoms suggestive of granulomatous disease affecting the upper and lower respiratory tract (radiograph showing fixed pulmonary infiltrates, nodules, or cavitations for >1 mo; bronchial stenosis; bloody nasal discharge and crusting for >1 mo or nasal ulceration; chronic sinusitis, otitis media, or mastoiditis for >3 mo; retro-orbital mass or inflammation [pseudotumor]; subglottic stenosis; saddle nose deformity/destructive sinonasal disease). [b] Surrogate markers for renal vasculitis (glomerulonephritis) are either hematuria associated with red cell casts or greater than 10% dysmorphic erythrocytes; or 2+ hematuria and 2+ proteinuria on urinalysis. (*Data from* Watts R, Lane S, Hanslik T, et al. Development and validation of a consensus methodology for the classification of the ANCA-associated vasculitides and PAN for epidemiological studies. Ann Rheum Dis 2007;66(2):222–7.)

Table 2
Clinical manifestations of PAN

Manifestation	Description	Frequency (%)
General symptoms	Fever, malaise, weight loss, arthralgias, myalgias	90
Neurologic	Mononeuritis multiplex, peripheral neuropathy	75
Cutaneous	Nodules, purpura, livedo	60
Renal	Increased creatinine level, hypertension, hematuria, proteinuria	50
Gastrointestinal	Abdominal pain, rectal bleeding	40
Orchitis	Testicular pain, swelling	20
Other		<10
Ophthalmologic	Retinal vasculitis/exudates, conjunctivitis, keratitis, uveitis	8
Vascular manifestations	Claudication, ischemia, necrosis	6
Cardiac	Cardiomyopathy, pericarditis	5
Central nervous system	Stroke, confusion	5
Respiratory	Lung infiltrates, pleural effusions	3

Data from Pagnoux C, Seror R, Henegar C, et al. Clinical features and outcomes in 348 patients with polyarteritis nodosa: a systematic retrospective study of patients diagnosed between 1963 and 2005 and entered into the French Vasculitis Study Group Database. Arthritis Rheum 2010;62(2):616–26.

system and skin are the most frequently involved territories.[27] Mononeuritis multiplex is the most common neurologic manifestation, although symmetric peripheral neuropathy also occurs.[28] Central nervous system involvement is rare.[27] Cutaneous features include purpura, livedoid lesions, subcutaneous nodules, and necrotic ulcers.[4] Limb edema is common.[27]

Organ ischemia, resulting from malperfusion from visceral microaneurysmal disease and associated arterial branch occlusion, is the most profound and disabling manifestation of the disease. The kidneys are the most common internal organ affected, with tissue infarction and hematomas usually produced by renal microaneurysm ischemia and rupture.[29] Kidney infarcts can be clinically silent or can produce hematuria and proteinuria.[29] PAN does not result in glomerulonephritis. New onset hypertension secondary to intrarenal artery involvement occurs in up to 35% of patients.[27] Kidney function is usually spared but multiple renal infarcts or uncontrolled hypertension may decrease renal function.[29] PAN has a striking tendency to spare the lungs, as opposed to other ANCA-associated vasculitis, such as MPA and granulomatosis with polyangiitis (Wegener) (GPA), which frequently involve the lungs and kidneys.

Laboratory Features

There are no laboratory abnormalities specific for PAN. Acute phase reactants, such as erythrocyte sedimentation rate and C-reactive protein, are commonly increased.[27] Chronic anemia is also frequently present.[27] Serologies for HBV, HCV, and HIV are usefully for diagnosing viral-associated PAN.[3] Cryoglobulins are characteristically negative and complement consumption, such as typical in cryoglobulinemic vasculitis, is unusual. ANCA is typically negative and their presence strongly points toward other systemic vasculitides, such as MPA, GPA, or eosinophilic GPA (Churg-Strauss).[10]

Histopathology

Histopathologic evidence of vascular inflammation in medium-sized or small arteries is crucial to the diagnosis of PAN.[8,10] Biopsies of symptomatic sites should be performed, and when many organs are involved, the less aggressive approach is preferable (ie, skin, muscle, sural nerve). Combined muscle and nerve biopsies in symptomatic patients have been shown to provide confirmation of PAN in up to 80% of patients, and muscle biopsies alone showed vascular inflammation in 65% in these patients.[27] Blind muscle and nerve biopsies show vasculitis in up to one-third of cases.[2] Testicular biopsies were advised in the past based on the frequency of involvement in PAN, but blind testicular biopsies are not currently recommended.[30] Testicular biopsies should be performed only when the testes are clinically involved or biopsies from other symptomatic sites have been negative. Because of the potential for hemorrhage from microaneurysms, ultrasound-controlled kidney and liver biopsies should be performed only if other approaches have been unsuccessful.

Vascular lesions in PAN are typically segmental and occur in branching points (**Fig. 2**). The inflammatory infiltrates are usually mixed and include neutrophils, lymphocytes, and macrophages.[31] Giant cells and granulomas are typically absent.[2] Fibrinoid necrosis is seen with early and active lesions, with neutrophil predominance.[31] Later stages usually show lymphocyte and macrophage infiltration along with neoangiogenesis.[31] Advanced lesions show intimal hyperplasia and fibrotic changes.[31] Inflammation of the blood vessels may result in the formation of microaneurysms and thrombosis. Vessels with different stages of the inflammatory process coexisting, including fibrinoid necrosis and fibrosis, is typical of PAN.[31]

Radiographic Features

Angiography of the viscera (particularly abdominal, renal, or cardiac arteries) can be performed when PAN is suspected and biopsy cannot be achieved. Typical lesions show multiple aneurysms (1–5 mm in diameter), usually coexisting with stenotic lesions, predominantly in kidney, mesenteric, and hepatic artery branches.[2] Renal infarctions can be seen but are not specific for PAN. Less invasive arteriography techniques, such as computed tomography and magnetic resonance imaging, can also be used. If histopathology cannot be obtained, a diagnosis of PAN can be established if typical radiographic abnormalities are present.[13] These techniques can establish the extent of the disease in PAN and track the disease course and treatment response.

Subsets of PAN

Cutaneous PAN

cPAN is a rare subset of PAN that lacks significant internal organ involvement. cPAN usually appears first as livedo reticularis, tender subcutaneous nodules, or cutaneous ulcerations.[4] Other findings include petechiae, purpura, cutaneous necrosis, and even autoamputation. Lesions most commonly occur on the legs, followed by the arms and then the trunk.[32] Constitutional symptoms have been reported in up to 30% of patients.[33] The course is usually relapsing, remitting, and benign, lasting months to several years. Relapses are typical, lasting 2 to 8 weeks, although remission may occur after a course of steroids. The progression to systemic PAN is rare. Deep incisional skin biopsy including the subcutaneous tissue confirms the diagnosis.[4]

Single-organ disease

Occasionally, localized PAN lesions are discovered in surgical specimens, such as the appendix, gallbladder, testes, and other internal organs.[34] An extensive evaluation must be performed to exclude systemic disease. Regular clinical follow-up is

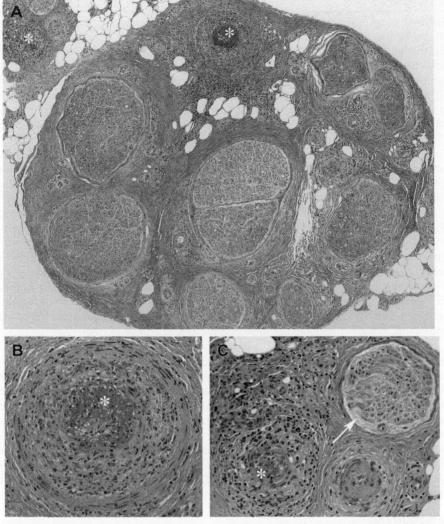

Fig. 2. A sural nerve from a patient symptomatically involved by mononeuritis multiplex in the setting of PAN. Histologic examination shows segmental involvement of medium-sized arteries (*asterisks*) with skip lesions. In the acute phase of the disease, the vessels are nearly or totally occluded by mixed inflammatory infiltrates containing neutrophils, lymphocytes, and monocytes and are associated with intramural fibrin deposits (bright red amorphous material). Associated nerve fascicles show subperineurial edema (*arrow* on C) and Wallerian degeneration of axons (original magnifications, ×100 [A], ×200 [B and C]).

important to determine if other anatomic areas have developed PAN or other clinical features are present or developing. In cases in which truly focal forms of PAN exist, excision is usually curative.[2]

Viral-associated PAN

Although HBV-PAN is virtually indistinguishable from classic PAN clinically, there are some differences among the viral-associated PAN entities (**Table 3**).[20,35–37] In

Table 3
Differences between viral-associated PAN

	HBV-PAN	HCV-PAN	HIV-PAN
Presentation	Waxing, waning	Acute	Acute
Time to symptom onset	6 mo (<1 y)	20 y	—
Viral characteristics	High levels of viral replication (high serum HBV DNA) and HBV antigen positivity	Not related to genotype or viral load	No specific relation to viral load
Age and sex	<40 y	Older women	—
Organs involved	Renal, gastrointestinal tract, central nervous system, skin	Skin most common (purpura), other organs same as HBV	Skin, joints, peripheral nerves and muscles
Severity	Severe	Moderate	Mild
Relapses	Common before treatment improvements, now rare (<10%)	Very common	Uncommon
Prognosis	Poor (35% mortality)	Fair (10% mortality)	Excellent
Response to therapy	Very good	Good	Excellent

Data from Patel N, Patel N, Khan T, et al. HIV infection and clinical spectrum of associated vasculitides. Curr Rheumatol Rep 2011;13(6):506–12.

addition, HBV-PAN has a greater frequency of gastrointestinal disorders, orchitis-like testicular disorders, severe arterial hypertension, and renal infarction compared with classic PAN and occurs more often in individuals younger than 40 years.[3,38] Hepatitis is rarely diagnosed first, because it remains mostly silent before PAN becomes clinically apparent.[3]

HCV seropositivity has been reported in patients with PAN, and in an international study of more than 1000 patients with hepatitis C, 7.6% were found to have PAN.[39,40] PAN is also believed to be the most common form of HIV-associated vasculitis, although it is still a rare entity.[3] Testing for HBV, HCV, and HIV in patients suspected of PAN is important, because they have consequences for treatment.[20]

DIFFERENTIAL DIAGNOSIS

The differential diagnosis of PAN is broad and includes infectious diseases and other entities that affect the vasculature and can cause arterial embolism, thrombosis, or vasospasm. Subacute bacterial endocarditis (including mycotic aneurysms with distal embolization), as well as HBV, HCV, and HIV, are among the infectious diseases that can mimic vasculitis or cause vascular inflammation.[3,20,35–37] Atherosclerosis, embolic disease from atrial myxomas or cholesterol deposits, segmental arteriolysis medial, calciphylaxis lesions, thrombotic disorders (antiphospholipid syndrome), fibromuscular dysplasia, and ergot use can mimic vasculitis of medium-sized arteries.[41,42] If disease affects the central nervous system, Moyamoya disease, MELAS (mitochondrial encephalomyopathy, lactic acidosis, and strokelike episodes), CADASIL (cerebral autosomal-dominant arteriopathy with subcortical infarcts and leukoencephalopathy), and granulomatous angiitis of the central nervous system are considerations. In children, Kawasaki disease affects medium-sized blood vessels, in particular the coronary arteries. Mononeuropathy multiplex can occur in diabetics, as well as other forms of systemic vasculitis, such as AAV and mixed cryoglobulinemia. Glomerulonephritis is much more typical of AAV.

TREATMENT

There are limited randomized controlled trial data supporting therapeutic decisions in PAN. Most studies were performed on mixed cohorts of patients with PAN and AAV.[43] The extent of organ involvement and disease progression guides treatment in PAN.

In an effort to study prognostic factors for PAN and other vasculitides, the FVSG developed the Five-Factor Score (FFS) in 1996 (**Table 4**).[44] Through multivariate analysis, they determined that the presence of certain factors could predict mortality. A 46% 5-year mortality was observed in patients with an FFS of 2 and 12% mortality in patients with a score of 0.[44] This score was revised in 2011 and includes only 4 factors, with the original score including central nervous systemic disease and proteinuria but not age (see **Table 4**).[45] This score is used to predict prognosis as well as guide treatment strategies.

If PAN is not associated with a viral syndrome, treatment relies mostly on corticosteroid therapy. Patients with mild PAN (FFS 0) and cPAN are usually treated with corticosteroids only, typically prednisone at about 1 mg/kg/d with subsequent tapering once remission is achieved. First-line corticosteroid therapy is able to achieve and maintain remission in about 50% of patients with mild PAN.[46]

If tapering is unsuccessful (prednisone <20 mg daily), if remission cannot be obtained, or if adverse effects of continued corticosteroid use are unacceptable in patients with mild PAN, methotrexate (MTX) (20–25 mg weekly) or azathioprine (AZA) (2 mg/kg/d) can be added.[46] MTX is faster acting but should be avoided in patients with renal and hepatic disease. In patients who are intolerant or have a contraindication to MTX or AZA, mycophenolate mofetil (2000–3000 mg daily) can be used.[46] The choice of agent depends on individual toxicity profiles and patient and physician preference.

For patients with FFS of 1 or greater, immunosuppressive agents are given in addition to prednisone. Cyclophosphamide (CYC) is used as 2 mg/kg/d orally or intravenous infusions (every 2 weeks for 3 doses, then monthly) at 0.6 g/m² for 4 to 12 months.[47,48] Monthly pulse CYC is preferred over daily oral CYC because of a better observed safety profile in PAN.[43,47] Remission agents, such as AZA and MTX, are advised once remission is achieved for a total duration of 18 months, mostly

Table 4
The FFS for PAN

FFS		Revised FFS	
Factors Predicting Mortality	**Points**	**Factors Predicting Mortality**	**Points**
Renal insufficiency (serum creatinine level >1.58 mg/dL)	1	Renal insufficiency (serum creatinine level >1.7 mg/dL)	1
Proteinuria >1 g/d	1		
Gastrointestinal involvement	1	Gastrointestinal involvement	1
Cardiac involvement	1	Cardiac involvement	1
Neurologic involvement	1	Age >65 y	1

Data from Guillevin L, Lhote F, Gayraud M, et al. Prognostic factors in polyarteritis nodosa and Churg-Strauss syndrome. A prospective study in 342 patients. Medicine (Baltimore) 1996;75(1):17–28; and Guillevin L, Pagnoux C, Seror R, et al. The Five-Factor Score revisited: assessment of prognoses of systemic necrotizing vasculitides based on the French Vasculitis Study Group (FVSG) cohort. Medicine (Baltimore) 2001;90:19.

borrowed from evidence from trials performed in patients with AAV.[49] CYC should not be used for more than 12 months.

Pulse steroid therapy can be initiated in patients with severe organ-threatening or life-threatening involvement or progression of mononeuritis multiplex. None of the data support first-line plasmapheresis in PAN unrelated to hepatitis viruses, even in patients with poor prognosis. However, plasmapheresis can be helpful in refractory PAN cases.[50,51] Surgery may be required for some disease complications, such as perforation, ischemia, or hemorrhage of internal organs (ie, gastrointestinal tract or kidneys).

For many years, HBV-PAN was treated like nonviral PAN and patients received corticosteroids and immunosuppressive agents, such as CYC. This regimen seemed to promote viral persistence and replication, thereby increasing the risk of chronic hepatitis and cirrhosis, and is no longer recommended.[21,50] In patients with mild PAN and evidence of infection with HBV, antivirals (lamivudine or interferon α) should be used as first-line therapy. Some patients with moderate to severe PAN with HBV infection may benefit from a short course of corticosteroids (1 week of prednisone 1 mg/kg/d, with subsequent tapering over the following week) along with plasmapheresis until antiviral therapy becomes effective.[20] The overall goal is to obtain HBV seroconversion (HBV e antigen to antibody), because once seroconversion is obtained, patients usually maintain complete remission without relapse. This process has been observed in about half of those patients with HBV-PAN treated with antiviral therapy.[3]

Large series describing treatment approaches for HCV-PAN and HIV-PAN have not been reported. Mild PAN cases associated with HCV and HIV should be treated with antiviral therapy.[35–37] Treatment of moderate to severe HCV-PAN has been adapted from the approach followed in HCV-associated cryoglobulinemic vasculitis, consisting of antiviral therapy (pegylated interferon α and ribavirin) along with immunosuppressive therapy (corticosteroids, CYC, or rituximab).[37] HIV-associated PAN seems to have an excellent response to treatment, using mostly moderate dose steroids (about 0.5 mg/kg/d) with concomitant highly active antiretroviral therapy, with rare use of cytotoxics.[35] PAN associated with parvovirus is rare but can respond to intravenous immunoglobulin therapy.[50]

PROGNOSIS

Untreated PAN has a poor prognosis, with a 13% 5-year survival rate.[27] Treatment of PAN has improved prognosis, with a 5-year survival rate of approximately 80%.[27] The survival rates for patients with HBV-PAN are lower than for patients with non–HBV-associated disease. The 5-year mortality of HBV-PAN has been reported to be 35%, but whether the prognosis of HBV-associated PAN has improved with the introduction of newer antiviral treatments is unknown.[3] Survival is better among those with cutaneous disease and limited organ involvement.

FUTURE CONSIDERATIONS/SUMMARY

As vasculitis definitions evolve, knowledge increases, and key triggers such as HBV decline, PAN has become a rare disease. International efforts are under way to better define and treat this disease.

REFERENCES

1. Wu W, Chaer RA. Nonarteriosclerotic vascular disease. Surg Clin North Am 2013; 93:833–75.

2. Hernández-Rodríguez J, Alba MA, Prieto-González S, et al. Diagnosis and classification of polyarteritis nodosa. J Autoimmun 2014;48–49:84–9.

3. Guillevin L. Infections in vasculitis. Best Pract Res Clin Rheumatol 2013;27(1): 19–31.

4. Morgan AJ, Schwartz RA. Cutaneous polyarteritis nodosa: a comprehensive review. Int J Dermatol 2010;49(7):750–6.

5. Kussmaul A, Maier R. Ueber eine bisher nicht beschriebene eigenthumliche arterienerkrankung (Periarteritis nodosa), die mit morbus brightii und rapid fortschreitender allgemeiner Muskellahmung einhergeht. Dtsch Arch Klin Med 1866;1:484–518 [in German].

6. Lightfoot RW Jr, Michel BA, Bloch DA, et al. The American College of Rheumatology 1990 criteria for the classification of polyarteritis nodosa. Arthritis Rheum 1990;33(8):1088–93.

7. Rao JK, Allen NB, Pincus T. Limitations of the 1990 American College of Rheumatology classification criteria in the diagnosis of vasculitis. Ann Intern Med 1998; 129(5):345–52.

8. Jennette JC, Falk RJ, Andrassy K, et al. Nomenclature of systemic vasculitides. Proposal of an International Consensus Conference. Arthritis Rheum 1994;37: 187–92.

9. Guillevin L, Lhote F, Amouroux J, et al. Antineutrophil cytoplasmic antibodies, abnormal angiograms and pathological findings in polyarteritis nodosa and Churg-Strauss syndrome: indications for the classification of vasculitides of the polyarteritis Nodosa Group. Br J Rheumatol 1996;35(10):958–64.

10. Jennette JC, Falk RJ, Bacon PA, et al. 2012 revised International Chapel Hill Consensus Conference nomenclature of vasculitides. Arthritis Rheum 2013; 65(1):1–11.

11. Lane SE, Watts RA, Barker TH, et al. Evaluation of the Sørensen diagnostic criteria in the classification of systemic vasculitis. Rheumatology (Oxford) 2002; 41(10):1138–41.

12. Bruce IN, Bell AL. A comparison of two nomenclature systems for primary systemic vasculitis. Br J Rheumatol 1997;36(4):453–8.

13. Watts R, Lane S, Hanslik T, et al. Development and validation of a consensus methodology for the classification of the ANCA-associated vasculitides and polyarteritis nodosa for epidemiological studies. Ann Rheum Dis 2007;66(2):222–7.

14. Liu LJ, Chen M, Yu F, et al. Evaluation of a new algorithm in classification of systemic vasculitis. Rheumatology (Oxford) 2008;47(5):708–12.

15. Henegar C, Pagnoux C, Puéchal X, et al. A paradigm of diagnostic criteria for polyarteritis nodosa: analysis of a series of 949 patients with vasculitides. Arthritis Rheum 2008;58(5):1528–38. Available at: http://www.ncbi.nlm.nih.gov/pubmed/?term=A+Paradigm+of+Diagnostic+Criteria+for+Polyarteritis+Nodosa+Analysis+of+a+Series+of+949+Patients+With+Vasculitides.

16. Luqmani RA, Suppiah R, Grayson PC, et al. Nomenclature and classification of vasculitis– update on the ACR/EULAR diagnosis and classification of vasculitis study (DCVAS). Clin Exp Immunol 2011;164(Suppl 1):11–3.

17. Craven A, Robson J, Ponte C, et al. ACR/EULAR-endorsed study to develop diagnostic and classification criteria for vasculitis (DCVAS). Clin Exp Nephrol 2013;17(5):619–21.

18. Watts RA, Lane SE, Bentham G, et al. Epidemiology of systemic vasculitis: a ten-year study in the United Kingdom. Arthritis Rheum 2000;43(2):414–9.

19. Ozen S, Pistorio A, Iusan SM, et al. EULAR/PRINTO/PRES criteria for Henoch-Schönlein purpura, childhood polyarteritis nodosa, childhood Wegener

granulomatosis and childhood Takayasu arteritis: Ankara 2008. Part II: final classification criteria. Ann Rheum Dis 2010;69(5):798–806.

20. Kallenberg CG, Tadema H. Vasculitis and infections: contribution to the issue of autoimmunity reviews devoted to "autoimmunity and infection". Autoimmun Rev 2008;8(1):29–32.

21. Trepo C, Guillevin L. Polyarteritis nodosa and extrahepatic manifestations of HBV infection: the case against autoimmune intervention in pathogenesis. J Autoimmun 2001;16(3):269–74.

22. Mahr A, Guillevin L, Poissonnet M, et al. Prevalences of polyarteritis nodosa, microscopic polyangiitis, Wegener's granulomatosis, and Churg-Strauss syndrome in a French urban multiethnic population in 2000: a capture-recapture estimate. Arthritis Rheum 2004;51(1):92–9.

23. Mohammad AJ, Jacobsson LT, Mahr AD, et al. Prevalence of Wegener's granulomatosis, microscopic polyangiitis, polyarteritis nodosa and Churg-Strauss syndrome within a defined population in Southern Sweden. Rheumatology (Oxford) 2007;46(8):1329–37.

24. Ormerod AS, Cook MC. Epidemiology of primary systemic vasculitis in the Australian Capital Territory and south-eastern New South Wales. Intern Med J 2008;38(11):816–23.

25. Selga D, Mohammad A, Sturfelt G, et al. Polyarteritis nodosa when applying the Chapel Hill nomenclature–a descriptive study on ten patients. Rheumatology 2006;45:1276–81.

26. Elkan PN, Pierce SB, Segel R, et al. Mutant adenosine deaminase 2 in a polyarteritis nodosa vasculopathy. N Engl J Med 2014;370(10):921–31.

27. Pagnoux C, Seror R, Henegar C, et al. Clinical features and outcomes in 348 patients with polyarteritis nodosa: a systematic retrospective study of patients diagnosed between 1963 and 2005 and entered into the French Vasculitis Study Group Database. Arthritis Rheum 2010;62(2):616–26.

28. Minegar A, Fowler M, Harris M, et al. Neurologic presentations of systemic vasculitides. Neurol Clin 2010;28:171–84.

29. El-Reshaid K, Kapoor MM, El-Reshaid W, et al. The spectrum of renal disease associated with microscopic polyangiitis and classic polyarteritis nodosa in Kuwait. Nephrol Dial Transplant 1997;12(9):1874–82.

30. Albert DA, Rimon D, Silverstein MD. The diagnosis of polyarteritis nodosa. I. A literature-based decision analysis approach. Arthritis Rheum 1988;31(9): 1117–27.

31. Cid MC, Grau JM, Casademont J, et al. Immunohistochemical characterization of inflammatory cells and immunologic activation markers in muscle and nerve biopsy specimens from patients with systemic polyarteritis nodosa. Arthritis Rheum 1994;37(7):1955061.

32. Marzano A, Vezzoli P, Berti E. Skin involvement in cutaneous and systemic vasculitis. Autoimmun Rev 2013;12:467–76.

33. Hoffman M. Atypical ulcers. Dermatol Ther 2013;26:222–35.

34. Hernández-Rodríguez J, Hoffman GS. Updating single-organ vasculitis. Curr Opin Rheumatol 2012;24(1):38–45.

35. Patel N, Patel N, Khan T, et al. HIV infection and clinical spectrum of associated vasculitides. Curr Rheumatol Rep 2011;13(6):506–12.

36. Pipitone N, Salvarani C. The role of infectious agents in the pathogenesis of vasculitis. Best Pract Res Clin Rheumatol 2008;22(5):897–911.

37. Saadoun D, Terrier B, Semoun O, et al. Hepatitis C virus-associated polyarteritis nodosa. Arthritis Care Res (Hoboken) 2011;63(3):427–35.

38. Cacoub P, Terrier B. Hepatitis B-related autoimmune manifestations. Rheum Dis Clin North Am 2009;35(1):125–37.
39. Ferri C, Sebastiani M, Antonelli A, et al. Current treatment of hepatitis C-associated rheumatic diseases. Arthritis Res Ther 2012;14(3):215.
40. Ramos-Casals M, Muñoz S, Medina F, et al. Systemic autoimmune diseases in patients with hepatitis C virus infection: characterization of 1020 cases (The HISPAMEC Registry). J Rheumatol 2009;36(7):1442–8.
41. Pontes Tde C, Rufino GP, Gurgel MG, et al. Fibromuscular dysplasia: a differential diagnosis of vasculitis. Rev Bras Reumatol 2012;52(1):70–4.
42. Filippone EJ, Foy A, Galanis T, et al. Segmental arterial mediolysis: report of 2 cases and review of the literature. Am J Kidney Dis 2011;58(6):981–7.
43. Adu D, Pall A, Luqmani RA, et al. Controlled trial of pulse versus continuous prednisolone and cyclophosphamide in the treatment of systemic vasculitis. QJM 1997;90(6):401–9.
44. Guillevin L, Lhote F, Gayraud M, et al. Prognostic factors in polyarteritis nodosa and Churg-Strauss syndrome. A prospective study in 342 patients. Medicine (Baltimore) 1996;75(1):17–28.
45. Guillevin L, Pagnoux C, Seror R, et al. The Five-Factor Score revisited: assessment of prognoses of systemic necrotizing vasculitides based on the French Vasculitis Study Group (FVSG) cohort. Medicine (Baltimore) 2011;90:19.
46. Ribi C, Cohen P, Pagnoux C, et al. Treatment of polyarteritis nodosa and microscopic polyangiitis without poor-prognosis factors: a prospective randomized study of one hundred twenty-four patients. Arthritis Rheum 2010;62(4):1186–97.
47. Gayraud M, Guillevin L, Cohen P, et al. Treatment of good-prognosis polyarteritis nodosa and Churg-Strauss syndrome: comparison of steroids and oral or pulse cyclophosphamide in 25 patients. French Cooperative Study Group for Vasculitides. Br J Rheumatol 1997;36(12):1290–7.
48. Guillevin L, Cohen P, Mahr A, et al. Treatment of polyarteritis nodosa and microscopic polyangiitis with poor prognosis factors: a prospective trial comparing glucocorticoids and six or twelve cyclophosphamide pulses in sixty-five patients. Arthritis Rheum 2003;49(1):93–100.
49. Pagnoux C, Mahr A, Hamidou MA, et al. Azathioprine or methotrexate for maintenance of ANCA-associated vasculitis. N Engl J Med 2008;359(26):2790–803.
50. Puéchal X, Guillevin L. Therapeutic immunomodulation in systemic vasculitis: taking stock. Joint Bone Spine 2013;80(4):374–9.
51. Guillevin L, Pagnoux C. Indication for plasma exchange for systemic necrotizing vasculidities. Transfus Apher Sci 2007;36(2):179–85.

Primary Angiitis of the Central Nervous System in Adults and Children

Alicia Rodriguez-Pla, MD, PhD, MPH, Paul A. Monach, MD, PhD*

KEYWORDS

- Primary angiitis of the central nervous system • PACNS • cPACNS • CNS vasculitis
- Vasculitis

KEY POINTS

- The prognosis of both adult and childhood primary angiitis of the central nervous systems has improved with prompt and aggressive treatment.
- Classification into subtypes remains a work in progress, primarily because of the lack of knowledge about pathogenesis.
- Cyclophosphamide and glucocorticoids remain the usual therapeutic approach, but less toxic regimens are appropriate for some patients and are a major goal for future research.

INTRODUCTION

Central nervous system (CNS) vasculitis comprises a broad spectrum of disorders that result in inflammation and destruction of the blood vessels of the brain, spinal cord, and meninges. Primary CNS vasculitis, also known as primary angiitis of the CNS (PACNS), is confined to the CNS. CNS vasculitis is considered secondary when it occurs in the context of a multisystem inflammatory disease, such as a systemic vasculitis or lupus, or an infection, such as by varicella zoster virus.

PACNS was first considered a distinct clinical entity in 1959 by Cravioto and Feigin,[1] who described several cases of noninfectious granulomatous angiitis associated with the nervous system. The prognosis was considered grim until 1983, when Cupps and colleagues[2] reported successful treatment with a combination of cyclophosphamide and glucocorticoids, which resulted in enthusiasm for the prospect of good outcomes with early diagnosis and aggressive treatment.[3] It is considered a rare disease, although the number of reported cases has increased substantially with increased awareness.

Disclosure: The authors have nothing to disclose.
Section of Rheumatology, Department of Medicine, Boston University School of Medicine, 72 East Concord Street, E533, Boston, MA 02118, USA
* Corresponding author.
E-mail address: pmonach@bu.edu

Rheum Dis Clin N Am 41 (2015) 47–62
http://dx.doi.org/10.1016/j.rdc.2014.09.004
0889-857X/15/$ – see front matter Published by Elsevier Inc.

rheumatic.theclinics.com

CNS vasculitis is increasingly being recognized in children.[4] Similar to what happens in adults, inflammation of the cerebral blood vessels in children may be idiopathic, which is known as childhood PACNS (cPACNS) and affects otherwise healthy children, or secondary, when it is related to an underlying infection, systemic inflammatory disease, drug, or malignancy. As with adult PACNS, the impact of untreated childhood PACNS may be severe, with less than 50% survival and long-term brain damage in greater than 50% of survivors. However, studies in recent years have suggested that early diagnosis and treatment improve morbidity and mortality.[5–11]

PACNS has been comprehensively reviewed recently by several of the groups that have led the field over the past 20 years, and readers are referred to those reviews for additional details and accompanying references to the primary literature.[7–9] This article includes key areas of consensus and disagreement and incorporates some recent primary literature of interest to practicing rheumatologists.

EPIDEMIOLOGY

The only population-based study of PACNS estimated an incidence of 2.4 cases per 100,000 person-years in Olmstead County, Minnesota.[10] Both men and women are affected, with either male or female predominance reported in different series.[10–12] The median age at diagnosis in adults is approximately 50 years.[10,11] Increased mortality has been linked to cerebral infarctions and involvement of larger arteries.

cPACNS is also rare, but the number of cases described has increased rapidly since its initial description in case series and recognition as a disease that may be distinct from adult PACNS. Thus, no incidence rate is available. Vasculitis may be an important cause of strokes in children.[13–15]

PATHOPHYSIOLOGY

The cause and pathogenesis of PACNS remain unknown. Neurologic manifestations of CNS vasculitis are a consequence of ischemia and infarction or intracranial hemorrhage.[11] Infarcts were observed in approximately 40% of patients, whereas intracranial hemorrhage was found in 12% of the cases, in a study of 131 cases diagnosed at Mayo Clinic over a 25-year period.[11] Ischemia and infarction are thought to result from a combination of vessel narrowing and obstruction caused by wall inflammation, increased coagulability provoked by inflammatory cytokines, and vasomotor tone dysfunction. Inflammation may also result in hemorrhage by debilitating the vascular wall.[11]

Little is known about the ultimate cause of PACNS. Because many infectious agents have been associated with CNS vasculitis,[7] and because of the predominance of granulomatous lesions in this vasculitis, infectious agents have been suggested as triggers in PACNS, as in many other types of vasculitis. However, this hypothesis has not been proved.[7,16]

HISTOPATHOLOGY

PACNS affects medium-sized arteries and small vessels, including arterioles, capillaries, and venules of the brain parenchyma and the leptomeninges. The distribution of the lesions is patchy. Granulomatous, lymphocytic, and necrotizing are the 3 main described histopathologic patterns in adults, and are thought to remain unchanged over time.[7]

Granulomatous vasculitis is the most common type, seen in approximately 58% of patients. It is characterized by a vasculocentric mononuclear inflammation and granulomas with multinucleated cells. β4-Amyloid deposition is seen in almost 50% of biopsy specimens with this pattern. Amyloid is rarely noted in specimens with nongranulomatous PACNS vasculitis.[7]

Lymphocytic vasculitis is the second most common pattern, observed in 28% of cases. It is characterized by a predominance of lymphocytic inflammation, with occasional presence of plasma cells and vessel destruction.[7] Lymphocytic vasculitis, with a predominant intramural and perivascular T-cell infiltrate of the small muscular arteries, arterioles, capillaries, and venues, is the typical histology in small vessel angiography-negative cPACNS.[9]

The least common pattern is necrotizing vasculitis, which is associated with intracranial hemorrhage. It is characterized by transmural fibrinoid necrosis (similar to what is seen in polyarteritis nodosa) and has been reported in 14% of cases. In some instances, necrotizing and granulomatous vasculitis can coexist.[7]

The spinal cord is involved in about 5% of patients, but rarely in the absence of brain involvement.[17]

CLINICAL FEATURES

The clinical features of PACNS are nonspecific, likely related to the patchy distribution of the vascular lesions, which further complicates the diagnostic process. The initial clinical presentation is heterogeneous. The onset may be abrupt, although it is usually gradual and progressive. Headache, altered cognition, and persistent neurologic deficits or strokes are the most common manifestations.[11,12] These 3 manifestations have been reported as the initial symptoms in approximately 65% of cases.[10,11]

Headache is the most common reported symptom, although it is only reported in about 60% of patients.[11] Headache may present with a variety of characteristics. However, it is typically described as subacute, insidious, and diffuse, whereas a sudden-onset thunderclap headache should raise suspicion for reversible cerebral vasoconstriction syndrome (RCVS).[3]

Strokes and transient ischemic attacks are common, occurring in 30% to 50% of patients.[3] Stroke usually affects many different vessels; presentation as a single stroke is uncommon.

Table 1 presents a summary of the main clinical manifestations observed in the 2 largest published series of adults with PACNS. Although limited conclusions can be made from fewer than 200 cases, and clinical features were reported differently in the two series, 2 observations can be made. First, focal neurologic deficits and strokes seem to predominate in patients with angiogram-confirmed PACNS, whereas altered cognition is more common in those with biopsy-proven vasculitis; these findings make sense in light of the noninflammatory syndromes of hemispheric stroke versus multi-infarct dementia. Second, the differences between these series (such as gender distribution, visual disturbances, and constitutional symptoms) indicate that more case series in PACNS are needed, that approaches to considering this diagnosis and excluding other diagnoses may differ (note that 60%–70% of the cases in these articles were not biopsy proven), and that clinicians should be vigilant to the possibility of disease subtypes.

The clinical features in children with PACNS are similar to those in adults. The largest published series of cPACNS included a total of 62 patients with angiography-confirmed vasculitis, before angiography-negative cPACNS was fully defined.[18] There were 38 male patients, with a median age of 7.2 years. Focal neurologic deficits were the most frequent clinical symptoms, including acute hemiparesis in

Table 1
Main characteristics at diagnosis in the 2 largest cohorts of adult patients with PACNS

	Giannini et al,[11] 2012			de Boysson et al,[12] 2014		
	All Patients (n = 131)	Biopsy Confirmed (n = 41)	Angiogram Confirmed (n = 90)	All Patients (n = 52)	Biopsy Confirmed (n = 19)	Angiogram Confirmed (n = 33)
Male/Female	57/74	23/18	34/56	30/22	13/6	17/16
Age at diagnosis, median (range), y	48 (17/84)	58 (26-84)	47 (17-81)	43.5 (18-79)	42 (23-59)	46 (18-79)
Headache, n (%)	81 (62)	22 (54)	59 (66)	28 (54)	9 (47)	19 (58)
Cognitive impairment, n (%)	69 (53)	30 (73)	39 (43)	18 (35)	10 (53)	8 (24)
Focal neurologic deficit, n (%)	51 (39)	10 (24)	41 (46)	43 (83)	12 (63)	31 (94)
Speech disorders, n (%)	33 (25)	13 (31)	20 (22)	18 (35)	7 (37)	11 (33)
Ataxia, n (%)	23 (18)	5 (12)	18 (20)	6 (12)	2 (11)	4 (12)
Seizures, n (%)	22 (17)	7 (17)	15 (17)	17 (33)	11 (58)	6 (18)
Visual symptoms, n (%)	53 (41)	10 (24)	43 (48)	8 (15)	4 (21)	4 (12)
Constitutional symptoms,[a] n (%)	11 (8)	5 (12)	6 (7)	12 (23)	7 (16)	5 (15)

The names of the symptoms differed between the two articles, so the same symptoms may not have been captured in the same way. This table treats the following terms as synonymous: cognitive impairment and altered cognition. Focal neurologic deficit and persistent neurologic deficit or stroke. Speech disorders and aphasia. Ataxia and cerebellar ataxia. Giannini et al[11] also listed the following clinical findings: hemiparesis, transient ischemic attack, intracranial hemorrhage, amnestic syndrome, paresis, or quadriparesis. De Boysson et al[12] also listed vertigo and/or dizziness, impaired vigilance, dyskinesias, psychiatric disorders, and ear, nose, and throat symptoms.

[a] De Boysson listed fever and weight loss separately. This table lists the numbers for weight loss, which were higher than for fever; thus, these numbers probably understate the percentages of patients with constitutional symptoms in the study by De Boysson et al.[12]

80%, hemisensory deficit in 79%, and fine motor deficits in 73%. Diffuse neurologic deficits included concentration difficulties in 29% of patients, cognitive dysfunction in 37%, and mood/personality changes in 26%. Headaches were present in 56% and seizures in 15% of patients. Both headaches and seizures were much more frequent in children who had progressive disease than in those who showed a nonprogressive course (discussed later).[18]

DISEASE SUBTYPES
Primary Angiitis of the Central Nervous System in Adults

Several classification schemes have been proposed, but none of them has been universally accepted. The classification of PACNS into subtypes is challenging because little is known about the pathophysiology.

Three broad subtypes were described in the first effort: granulomatous angiitis of the CNS, benign angiopathy of the CNS (BACNS), and atypical PACNS.[19] More recently, BACNS has been recognized as a vasospastic disorder (renamed RCVS) and not vasculitis. Because of the heterogeneity in the atypical PACNS group, this term is now avoided.[8]

More recent approaches to classification have included different potential sources of heterogeneity:

1. Vessel size: biopsy-positive versus angiographically positive PACNS
2. Imaging (eg, mass lesion or leptomeningeal enhancement)
3. Clinical features (eg, rapidly progressive or hemorrhagic)
4. Histology: granulomatous, lymphocytic, amyloid, necrotizing

For example, Hajj-Ali and colleagues[8] recently proposed 5 subtypes based on available clinical, neuroimaging, angiographic, and pathologic data, whereas Salvarani and colleagues[7] initially proposed 6 and subsequently 7 subtypes[11] (**Table 2**).

Childhood Primary Angiitis of the Central Nervous System

Two major subtypes have been recognized in cPACNS: angiography-positive large vessel cPACNS and angiography-negative small vessel cPACNS. The angiography-positive subtype has been divided into 2 subcategories based on the course of the disease: progressive and nonprogressive large vessel cPACNS.[9] Among 62 children with angiography-confirmed vasculitis in the largest series, 20 (32%) had progressive cPACNS and 42 patients (68%) had the nonprogressive subtype.[18]

Table 2 Proposed disease subtypes in PACNS		
Adults		
Hajj-Ali et al,[8] 2011	**Salvarani et al,[7,11] 2012**	**Children[18]**
Granulomatous PACNS	Spinal cord abnormalities[7,11,17]	Angiography-positive
Lymphocytic PACNS[8,36]	Angiography-negative, biopsy-positive	large vessel cPACNS
Lymphocytic PACNS[8]	primary CNS vasculitis[7,11,21]	Nonprogressive cPACNS
Angiographically	Prominent leptomeningeal	Progressive cPACNS
defined PACNS[8,11,12]	enhancement on MRI[7,11,29]	Angiography-negative
Mass-lesion	Cerebral amyloid angiitis[7,11,43]	small vessel cPACNS
presentation[8,28]	Rapidly progressive PACNS[7,11,50]	
Amyloid β–related	Solitary tumorlike mass lesion[7,8,28]	
cerebral angiitis[8,49]	Intracranial hemorrhage[7,11,51]	

DIAGNOSIS

The possibility of CNS vasculitis is usually considered in 2 clinical settings: starting with either a constellation of symptoms or an abnormal angiogram. We propose 2 different diagnostic algorithms to approach a patient with clinical suspicion of PACNS (**Fig. 1**). Either way, it is a combination of symptoms, neurologic examination findings, cerebrospinal fluid (CSF) analysis, MRI, and angiography that leads to a decision whether to perform a brain biopsy, and whether to treat with immune-suppressive drugs even if such a biopsy is negative.

Laboratory Studies

There is no diagnostic laboratory study for PACNS. Results of blood tests in adults with PACNS are usually normal, including acute phase reactants, antinuclear antibodies, antineutrophil cytoplasm antibodies, and antiphospholipid antibodies.[10] Appropriate serologies, cultures, and molecular testing for pathogens that can cause infections mimicking PACNS are essential.[8,20]

CSF analysis is crucial for the assessment of patients with suspected PACNS, in order to address a broad differential diagnosis that includes infection or malignancy, and because normal CSF makes a diagnosis of PACNS less likely. Up to 90% of patients with biopsy-confirmed PACNS have abnormal CSF, although CSF may be normal in about 40% of patients with angiographically diagnosed disease.[8,12,20] Modest lymphocytic pleocytosis, normal glucose, and increased protein concentrations are frequently observed, and occasionally oligoclonal bands may be detected.[8,20] Patients with angiography-negative PACNS often have highly increased CSF protein levels.[21]

In children with nonprogressive angiography-positive large vessel cPACNS, the acute phase reactants in blood and the CSF analysis are usually within the normal range. In these children, CSF and serologic examination for evidence of varicella zoster virus infection should be performed.[9] In progressive angiography-positive large vessel cPACNS, the acute phase reactants are frequently normal as well, although a mild increase can also be observed. CSF analysis may be either normal or abnormal,

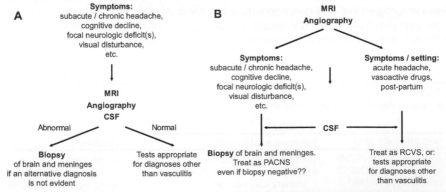

Fig. 1. Proposed diagnostic algorithms, based on the usual settings in which a rheumatologist is consulted about the possibility of PACNS. (*A*) The rheumatologist is consulted because of a symptom complex and usually after some imaging has been done. (*B*) The consult is based primarily on angiography and often with abnormalities on MRI as well: a setting in which RCVS is a particularly important alternative consideration based on the different symptoms from those of PACNS. CSF, cerebrospinal fluid.

revealing mild pleocytosis, increased protein, and/or increased opening pressure.[9,18] Children affected by angiography-negative small vessel vasculitis typically present with increased levels of inflammatory markers such as C-reactive protein, erythrocyte sedimentation rate, and C3.[6] Lymphocytic pleocytosis, increased protein levels, and/or increased opening pressure are frequently found in the CSF analysis.[6,9] Oligoclonal bands have been reported in one-third of the children with angiography-negative cPACNS.[6]

Electroencephalography

Most patients have mild, nonspecific electroencephalographic findings.[22]

Neuroimaging

MRI

MRI is the main neuroradiographic modality for the work-up of patients with suspected PACNS and has a sensitivity of 90% to 100%,[23] although poor specificity. The typical MRI abnormalities consist of changes in the subcortical white matter, deep gray and white matter, and the cerebral cortex.[24] Infarcts are the most common lesions, reported in 53% of patients in the largest series.[10] Multiple infarcts often occur.[25] Lesions in white matter identified with high-intensity T2-weighted MRI with a fluid-attenuated inversion recovery sequence are common but nonspecific, which makes it imperative to rule out other possible causes, including migraine, ischemic changes caused by noninflammatory vascular disease, demyelinating lesions, myelinolysis, metastasis, eclampsia, and changes secondary to neurometabolic diseases.[8,26,27]

Mass lesions occur in around 5% of patients,[28] gadolinium enhancement of the leptomeninges in 8%,[29] and gadolinium-enhanced intracranial lesions in one-third.[30]

The correlation between MRI and angiographic findings is not perfect. Some studies have shown that MRI can be abnormal with normal findings on angiography, which reflects the inadequate resolution for angiography for small vessel disease.[31]

High-resolution MRI of the vessel wall is an emerging tool for evaluating intracranial artery disease and has the advantage of defining vessel wall characteristics.[32] Although this technique is promising, larger studies are needed to validate the initial observations.

Magnetic resonance angiography and computed tomography angiography

Magnetic resonance angiography (MRA) and computed tomography angiography (CTA) are less invasive than cerebral angiography, but their resolution is often inadequate for detecting vasculitic changes in the arteries that are usually affected in PACNS. These studies are thus of little use in the diagnosis of PACNS.[33] In patients with abnormal MRI but normal MRA or CTA in the context of suggestive clinical history, cerebral angiography should be performed.[7]

Angiography

The typical angiographic finding of PACNS is known as beading, which consists of alternating areas of stenosis and dilatation. Multiple arteries of different sizes are usually affected, and disease is usually, but not always, bilateral.[34] Microaneurysms are infrequent.[7] Although these angiographic findings are considered characteristic of PACNS, they are not specific and are also commonly found in atherosclerosis, radiation vasculopathy, infection, and vasospasm (RCVS).[8]

The specificity of cerebral angiography for diagnosis of PACNS may be as low as 30%.[35] Thus, although cerebral angiography is considered the radiological gold standard for PACNS, its results should always be interpreted in the clinical context and the results of all other diagnostic tests.[7,8] The sensitivity of angiography is also imperfect: in one study, only 43% of angiograms were characteristic of vasculitis in patients with biopsy-proven CNS vasculitis,[10] and one leading group estimates the overall sensitivity of angiography for adult PACNS at 70%.[10]

Pathology

Although biopsy of brain or spinal cord is considered the gold standard to confirm the diagnosis of CNS vasculitis, the distribution of changes is often so focal and segmental that a biopsy may yield negative results in about 50% of cases.[2,8,36] The role of the biopsy is double: for identification of angiitis in cases in which vascular imaging is inconclusive and for ruling out mimics, especially infections and malignancy. Alrawi and colleagues[37] found a wide variety of alternative diagnoses in 24 of the 61 patients (39%) in whom a brain biopsy was performed specifically because of high suspicion for CNS vasculitis.

Several strategies may be adopted to increase the likelihood of obtaining a diagnostic biopsy, including targeting sites of imaging abnormality, combining parenchymal and leptomeningeal sampling, and choosing a biopsy site based on intraoperative appearance.[38] In the absence of a clear target lesion based on imaging, a blind biopsy has a very low yield.[38]

DIAGNOSTIC CRITERIA

Diagnostic criteria were proposed by Calabrese and Mallek[36] in 1988. These criteria were also adopted for cPACNS and, although they have never been validated for use in children or adults, they have been widely used in clinical practice and research[18]:

1. The presence of an acquired, otherwise unexplained neurologic or psychiatric manifestation
2. The presence of either classic angiographic or histopathologic features of angiitis within the CNS
3. No evidence of systemic vasculitis or any disorder that could cause or mimic the angiographic or pathologic features of the disease

To prevent misdiagnosis, especially with recognition of RCVS, Birnbaum and Hellmann[23] recently proposed to classify the patients with definite PACNS when biopsy confirmation was obtained and probable otherwise.

DIFFERENTIAL DIAGNOSIS

The differential diagnosis of PACNS is extensive. Many other disorders (most of them probably even less common than PACNS) can mimic PACNS, so careful medical assessment is recommended to rule them out to avoid therapeutic and prognostic errors (**Box 1**).[7,8,33]

By far the most common mimicker of PACNS, because of its similar angiographic appearance, is RCVS. In 2007, RCVS was proposed as a collective name for various disorders that are characterized by brain vasoconstriction rather than by vasculitis.[39]

Disease features that best allow distinction between PACNS and RCVS are shown in **Table 3**. The key clinical manifestation is recurrent thunderclap headache in 78% to 100% of cases. Neurologic deficits, either transient or persistent, occur in around 43% of cases, seizures in 17%. The headache can be precipitated by maneuvers that increase intracranial pressure. Serotonergic or adrenergic agents, recreational drugs, and postpartum state have been associated with RCVS in about 50% of patients.[3,40]

Box 1
Differential diagnosis of PACNS

- RCVS
  - Call-Fleming syndrome[a]
  - Postpartum angiopathy
  - Migrainous vasospasm
  - Drug-induced arteritis
  - BACNS
- Secondary CNS vasculitis
  - Infections
    - Bacterial
    - Viral
    - Mycoplasmal
    - Fungal
    - Protozoal
    - Rickettsial
  - Systemic vasculitides
    - Granulomatosis with polyangiitis (Wegener granulomatosis)
    - Polyarteritis nodosa
    - Eosinophilic granulomatosis with polyangiitis (Churg-Strauss syndrome)
    - Behçet disease
    - Henoch-Schönlein purpura
    - Kawasaki disease
    - Giant cell arteritis
    - Takayasu arteritis
    - Hypocomplementemic urticarial vasculitis
  - Systemic autoimmune and inflammatory diseases
    - Rheumatoid arthritis
    - Systemic lupus erythematosus
    - Dermatomyositis
    - Morphea or linear scleroderma
    - Cogan syndrome
    - Sarcoidosis
    - Inflammatory bowel disease
    - Sjögren syndrome
    - Autoinflammatory syndromes
- Nonvasculitic autoimmune and inflammatory brain diseases
  - N-Methyl-D-aspartate receptor–mediated encephalitis
  - Neuromyelitis optica
  - Susac syndrome[b]

- o Acute demyelinating encephalomyelitis
- o Optic neuritis
- o Multiple sclerosis
- o Rasmussen encephalitis[c]
- Other noninflammatory vasculopathies apart from RCVS
  - o Fibromuscular dysplasia
  - o Moyamoya disease[d]
  - o Intracranial dissection
  - o Radiation vasculopathy
  - o Rare inherited vasculopathies (eg, CADASIL[e])
- Miscellaneous
  - o Thromboembolic disease
  - o Bacterial endocarditis
  - o Antiphospholipid syndrome and other hypercoagulable states
  - o Cardiac myxoma embolism
  - o Cholesterol atheroembolism
  - o Angiotropic and intravascular lymphoproliferative disorders
  - o Hemoglobin disorders
  - o Malignancy-related angiitis (Hodgkin and non-Hodgkin lymphoma, leukemia, lung cancer)
  - o Graft-versus-host-reaction

This list encompasses entities with a wide range of incidence/prevalence, from common to extremely rare.

[a] Call-Fleming syndrome was first described in 1988 by Call and colleagues, when they described 19 patients with "reversible cerebral arterial segmental vasoconstriction," manifested with thunderclap headaches with or without focal neurologic symptoms and without evidence of subarachnoid hemorrhage. This syndrome and the others listed under RCVS are now thought to be the same disorder.[40]

[b] Susac syndrome, also known as retinocochleocerebral vasculopathy, is a microangiopathy of unknown cause first described by Dr John Susac in 1979 and characterized by encephalopathy, retinal artery occlusion, and hearing loss. It often presents with personality change and bizarre and paranoid behavior.[52]

[c] Rasmussen encephalitis, or chronic focal encephalitis, is a rare inflammatory neurologic disease, characterized by frequent and severe seizures, loss of motor skills and speech, hemiparesis, encephalitis, and dementia. It affects a single cerebral hemisphere and it generally affects children younger than 15 years. It is named for the neurosurgeon Theodore Rasmussen.[53]

[d] Moyamoya disease is a cerebrovascular disease of unknown cause characterized by progressive stenosis of the intracranial internal carotid arteries and their proximal branches. It generally affects adults in the third to fourth decade of life. In children it produces strokes or seizures. In adults it typically causes strokes, recurrent transient ischemic attacks, sensorimotor paralysis, seizures, and/or migrainelike headaches.[54]

[e] Cerebral autosomal dominant arteriopathy with subcortical infarcts and leukoencephalopathy (CADASIL) is a genetic disorder characterized by migraine and cumulative stroke and cognitive deficits. It typically manifests in young individuals with headache, stroke, and white matter changes on MRI.[8]

Data from Salvarani C, Brown RD Jr, Hunder GG. Adult primary central nervous system vasculitis. Lancet 2012;380(9843):767–77; and Hajj-Ali RA. Primary angiitis of the central nervous system: differential diagnosis and treatment. Best Pract Res Clin Rheumatol 2010;24(3):413–26.

Table 3
Main differences between PACNS and RCVS

	PACNS	RCVS
Gender	Similar (studies disagree)	Female
Mean age at onset (y)	~50	~40
Onset	More insidious onset	Acute
Clinical course	Progressive if untreated; monophasic or relapsing after treatment	Monophasic
Headache	Insidious: subacute or chronic	Acute onset, thunderclap
CSF findings	Lymphocytic pleocytosis and increased protein levels	Normal
Brain MRI	Abnormal in 90%–100%, ischemic, high-intensity T2/FLAIR lesions	Ischemia, edema, convexity subarachnoid hemorrhage, intracranial hemorrhage, but normal in 30%
Brain angiography	Normal in ~30%; stenoses or occlusions, usually multiple, often adjacent to dilatations; frequently irreversible	Abnormal in ~100% during the acute phase, not readily distinguishable from PACNS. Reversed after recovery
Brain biopsy	Vasculitis	No evidence of vasculitis
Treatment	Glucocorticoids, often combined with cytotoxic agents	Calcium channel blockers, particularly nimodipine

Abbreviations: FLAIR, fluid-attenuated inversion recovery; PACNS, primary angiitis of the central nervous system; RCVS, reversible cerebral vasoconstriction syndrome.
  Data from Refs.[7,20,40]

Diagnostic criteria of RCVS were proposed by Calabrese and colleagues.[39] Differentiation from PACNS is crucial because immunosuppressive therapy is not warranted for syndromes caused by vasoconstriction (see **Table 3**).[20]

MANAGEMENT
Treatment: Adult Primary Angiitis of the Central Nervous System

Treatment guidelines in adult PACNS are based on retrospective data and expert opinion because no controlled studies are available given the rarity of this condition.[3] The earliest reports suggested a poor outcome in most patients, and doubtful effectiveness of glucocorticoids alone.[7,41] Cupps and colleagues[2] reported the effectiveness of cyclophosphamide in combination with corticosteroids, and other studies corroborated their findings.[10,42]

Because it is impossible to predict accurately which patients would do well with less-aggressive regimens, it is always reasonable to treat with glucocorticoids and cyclophosphamide. However, it is also appropriate to base initial treatment on the severity of symptoms and imaging findings and to use a less-aggressive regimen for patients with milder disease,[7] analogous to the stratification that is typically used in the systemic vasculitides.[3] Patients with only small vessels affected (characterized by prominent leptomeningeal enhancement on MRI or by negative cerebral angiogram and a positive brain biopsy) are particularly likely to have a rapid response to treatment with a favorable neurologic outcome.[29,43] Whether the less-aggressive approach should mean glucocorticoids alone[7] or should routinely include azathioprine or myco-phenolate is unclear.[7,33]

Glucocorticoids should be started promptly. The recommended initial dose of pred-nisone is 1 mg/kg per day. Some experts advise giving intravenous pulse methylpred-nisolone for 3 days before switching to high-dose oral glucocorticoids.[7]

The usual oral dose of cyclophosphamide is 2 mg/kg daily and probably should be adjusted for age and renal dysfunction, as has been done in trials in the systemic vascu-litides. Intravenous pulses of cyclophosphamide for 6 months may be safer than daily oral therapy,[44] but no comparison of effectiveness in PACNS has been made. Once remission has been achieved after 3 to 6 months of treatment, cyclophosphamide is switched to azathioprine (1–2 mg/kg) or mycophenolate (1000–2000 mg/d)[3,7] rather than methotrexate, which does not penetrate the CNS well. The recommended duration of therapy is approximately 18 months,[7,10] assuming that relapses do not mandate prolonged treatment.

For the minority of patients who experience frequent relapses, there is no guideline for therapy, and efforts to maintain remission may include occasional steroid pulses and/or long-term use of azathioprine, mycophenolate, low-dose glucocorticoids, or biologics.[7]

Tumor necrosis factor (TNF) blockers have been reported anecdotally to be useful in 2 cases of PACNS,[45] and rituximab in 3 cases.[46,47] We suspect that the off-label use of biologics, particularly anti-TNF drugs and rituximab, extends well beyond the literature (eg, we have used anti-TNF drugs in 2 patients with recurrent PACNS), but no conclu-sions about their absolute or relative effectiveness can be drawn.

Treatment: Childhood Primary Angiitis of the Central Nervous System

Because of evidence that nonprogressive angiography-positive large vessel cPACNS is an inflammatory disease, glucocorticoids have been recommended in the acute phase of the illness.[9] Based on observational data suggesting improved neurologic outcomes, a 5-day course of intravenous methylprednisolone followed by 3 months of tapered oral glucocorticoids is an appropriate approach. Anticoagulation with heparin is also advised at presentation, followed by antiplatelet therapy.[9]

Treatment recommendations for progressive angiography-positive large vessel cPACNS include induction therapy with high-dose glucocorticoids and cyclophospha-mide for 6 months, followed by mycophenolate mofetil maintenance treatment for 18 months, and antithrombotic therapy.[9]

Angiography-negative small vessel cPACNS also requires aggressive treatment. Remission-induction with cyclophosphamide and high-dose glucocorticoids for 6 months led to complete neurologic recovery in 70% of children in one study.[6] The same nonrandomized study used an additional 18 months of maintenance therapy and suggested that mycophenolate mofetil was superior to azathioprine for preventing disease flares. Successful treatment with infliximab has been reported in 2 cases of refractory small vessel cPACNS.[48] In contrast with angiography-positive cPACNS, antithrombotic therapy has not been recommended for angiography-negative small vessel disease. Treatment to manage resulting seizure disorders and psychotic symp-toms is often needed.[9]

Monitoring Disease Activity

Along with careful neurologic examinations, serial MRI and MRA every 4 to 6 weeks early in the course of treatment, then every 3 to 4 months during the first year of treat-ment or when a new neurologic deficit arises, are useful to monitor disease course.[33] In patients with stable imaging but worsening clinical symptoms, repeat spinal fluid examination and repeat angiography may be necessary. For patients without biopsy verification at the time of initial diagnosis who have worsening symptoms despite therapy, a repeat brain biopsy should be considered.[7]

PROGNOSIS

Recurrences were recorded in only 26% to 27% of adult patients.[10–12] Patients with relapsing disease needed therapy for longer than did those with nonrelapsing disease, but otherwise had outcomes similar to those without relapses.[10]

Thus, treatment seems to be associated with a favorable outcome in most patients. In the Mayo series most patients with low disability at diagnosis continued to have low disability at last follow-up, and most of the 22 patients with severe disability at diagnosis had less, but still significant, disability at follow-up. These data emphasize the need for early diagnosis, because prompt treatment frequently leads to a favorable outcome.[10]

The long-term relapse risk and neurocognitive outcomes in cPACNS are not yet known.[9]

FUTURE CONSIDERATIONS

Although PACNS encompasses more uncertainties than certainties, authorities agree on the extent of that uncertainty and approach it in the same way, so there are no strong controversies in the field. Many unanswered questions remain about the pathogenesis of PACNS, and efficient noninvasive methods for diagnosis and evidence-based treatment guidelines are lacking. The most effective and safe regimen for cyclophosphamide and glucocorticoids is not well defined. Most importantly, it is not clear which patients need cyclophosphamide or whether other alternative medications would be as effective but safer.

Randomized trials of PACNS treatments are clearly needed, although recruitment will be challenging, and the possibility of disease subsets will need to be incorporated in the design and interpretation. Given the rarity of this condition, these trials require multicenter collaboration efforts. In advance of such studies, ongoing publication of case series[12] and even case reports[45–48] is still of considerable value.

REFERENCES

1. Cravioto H, Feigin I. Noninfectious granulomatous angiitis with a predilection for the nervous system. Neurology 1959;9:599–609.
2. Cupps TR, Moore PM, Fauci AS. Isolated angiitis of the central nervous system. Prospective diagnostic and therapeutic experience. Am J Med 1983;74(1): 97–105.
3. Hajj-Ali RA, Calabrese LH. Primary angiitis of the central nervous system. Autoimmun Rev 2013;12(4):463–6.
4. Cellucci T, Benseler SM. Central nervous system vasculitis in children. Curr Opin Rheumatol 2010;22(5):590–7.
5. Benseler SM, deVeber G, Hawkins C, et al. Angiography-negative primary central nervous system vasculitis in children: a newly recognized inflammatory central nervous system disease. Arthritis Rheum 2005;52(7):2159–67 [Papers of particular interest].
6. Hutchinson C, Elbers J, Halliday W, et al. Treatment of small vessel primary CNS vasculitis in children: an open-label cohort study. Lancet Neurol 2010;9(11): 1078–84.

7. Salvarani C, Brown RD Jr, Hunder GG. Adult primary central nervous system vasculitis. Lancet 2012;380(9843):767–77 [Papers of particular interest].

8. Hajj-Ali RA, Singhal AB, Benseler S, et al. Primary angiitis of the CNS. Lancet Neurol 2011;10(6):561–72 [Papers of particular interest].

9. Gowdie P, Twilt M, Benseler SM. Primary and secondary central nervous system vasculitis. J Child Neurol 2012;27(11):1448–59 [Papers of particular interest].

10. Salvarani C, Brown RD Jr, Calamia KT, et al. Primary central nervous system vasculitis: analysis of 101 patients. Ann Neurol 2007;62(5):442–51 [Papers of particular interest].

11. Giannini C, Salvarani C, Hunder G, et al. Primary central nervous system vasculitis: pathology and mechanisms. Acta Neuropathol 2012;123(6):759–72 [Papers of particular interest].

12. de Boysson H, Zuber M, Naggara O, et al. Primary angiitis of the central nervous system: description of the first fifty-two adults enrolled in the French cohort of patients with primary vasculitis of the central nervous system. Arthritis Rheumatol 2014;66(5):1315–26 [Papers of particular interest].

13. Gallagher KT, Shaham B, Reiff A, et al. Primary angiitis of the central nervous system in children: 5 cases. J Rheumatol 2001;28(3):616–23.

14. Lanthier S. Primary angiitis of the central nervous system in children: 10 cases proven by biopsy. J Rheumatol 2002;29(7):1575–6.

15. Moharir M, Shroff M, Benseler SM. Childhood central nervous system vasculitis. Neuroimaging Clin North Am 2013;23(2):293–308.

16. Arthur G, Margolis G. Mycoplasma-like structures in granulomatous angiitis of the central nervous system. Case reports with light and electron microscopic studies. Arch Pathol Lab Med 1977;101(7):382–7.

17. Salvarani C, Brown RD Jr, Calamia KT, et al. Primary CNS vasculitis with spinal cord involvement. Neurology 2008;70(24 Pt 2):2394–400.

18. Benseler SM, Silverman E, Aviv RI, et al. Primary central nervous system vasculitis in children. Arthritis Rheum 2006;54(4):1291–7.

19. Calabrese LH, Duna GF, Lie JT. Vasculitis in the central nervous system. Arthritis Rheum 1997;40(7):1189–201.

20. Hajj-Ali RA, Calabrese LH. Diagnosis and classification of central nervous system vasculitis. J Autoimmun 2014;48–49:149–52.

21. Kadkhodayan Y, Alreshaid A, Moran CJ, et al. Primary angiitis of the central nervous system at conventional angiography. Radiology 2004;233(3):878–82.

22. Salvarani C, Brown RD Jr, Hunder GG. Adult primary central nervous system vasculitis: an update. Curr Opin Rheumatol 2012;24(1):46–52.

23. Birnbaum J, Hellmann DB. Primary angiitis of the central nervous system. Arch Neurol 2009;66(6):704–9.

24. Pomper MG, Miller TJ, Stone JH, et al. CNS vasculitis in autoimmune disease: MR imaging findings and correlation with angiography. AJNR Am J Neuroradiol 1999; 20(1):75–85.

25. Hurst RW, Grossman RI. Neuroradiology of central nervous system vasculitis. Semin Neurol 1994;14(4):320–40.

26. Appenzeller S, Faria AV, Zanardi VA, et al. Vascular involvement of the central nervous system and systemic diseases: etiologies and MRI findings. Rheumatol Int 2008;28(12):1229–37.

27. Bekiesinska-Figatowska M. T2-hyperintense foci on brain MR imaging. Med Sci Monit 2004;10(Suppl 3):80–7.

28. Molloy ES, Singhal AB, Calabrese LH. Tumour-like mass lesion: an under-recognised presentation of primary angiitis of the central nervous system. Ann Rheum Dis 2008;67(12):1732–5.
29. Salvarani C, Brown RD Jr, Calamia KT, et al. Primary central nervous system vasculitis with prominent leptomeningeal enhancement: a subset with a benign outcome. Arthritis Rheum 2008;58(2):595–603.
30. Parisi JE, Moore PM. The role of biopsy in vasculitis of the central nervous system. Semin Neurol 1994;14(4):341–8.
31. Greenan TJ, Grossman RI, Goldberg HI. Cerebral vasculitis: MR imaging and angiographic correlation. Radiology 1992;182(1):65–72.
32. Obusez EC, Hui F, Hajj-Ali RA, et al. High-resolution MRI vessel wall imaging: spatial and temporal patterns of reversible cerebral vasoconstriction syndrome and central nervous system vasculitis. AJNR Am J Neuroradiol 2014;35(8): 1527–32.
33. Hajj-Ali RA. Primary angiitis of the central nervous system: differential diagnosis and treatment. Best Pract Res Clin Rheumatol 2010;24(3):413–26.
34. Alhalabi M, Moore PM. Serial angiography in isolated angiitis of the central nervous system. Neurology 1994;44(7):1221–6.
35. Duna GF, Calabrese LH. Limitations of invasive modalities in the diagnosis of primary angiitis of the central nervous system. J Rheumatol 1995;22(4): 662–7.
36. Calabrese LH, Mallek JA. Primary angiitis of the central nervous system. Report of 8 new cases, review of the literature, and proposal for diagnostic criteria. Medicine (Baltimore) 1988;67(1):20–39.
37. Alrawi A, Trobe JD, Blaivas M, et al. Brain biopsy in primary angiitis of the central nervous system. Neurology 1999;53(4):858–60.
38. Miller DV, Salvarani C, Hunder GG, et al. Biopsy findings in primary angiitis of the central nervous system. Am J Surg Pathol 2009;33(1):35–43.
39. Calabrese LH, Dodick DW, Schwedt TJ, et al. Narrative review: reversible cerebral vasoconstriction syndromes. Ann Intern Med 2007;146(1):34–44 [Papers of particular interest].
40. Singhal AB, Hajj-Ali RA, Topcuoglu MA, et al. Reversible cerebral vasoconstriction syndromes: analysis of 139 cases. Arch Neurol 2011;68(8):1005–12 [Papers of particular interest].
41. Moore PM. Diagnosis and management of isolated angiitis of the central nervous system. Neurology 1989;39(2 Pt 1):167–73.
42. Fauci AS, Haynes B, Katz P. The spectrum of vasculitis: clinical, pathologic, immunologic and therapeutic considerations. Ann Intern Med 1978;89(5 Pt 1): 660–76.
43. Salvarani C, Brown RD Jr, Calamia KT, et al. Angiography-negative primary central nervous system vasculitis: a syndrome involving small cerebral vessels. Medicine (Baltimore) 2008;87(5):264–71.
44. de Groot K, Harper L, Jayne DR, et al. Pulse versus daily oral cyclophosphamide for induction of remission in antineutrophil cytoplasmic antibody-associated vasculitis: a randomized trial. Ann Intern Med 2009;150(10):670–80.
45. Salvarani C, Brown RD Jr, Calamia KT, et al. Efficacy of tumor necrosis factor alpha blockade in primary central nervous system vasculitis resistant to immunosuppressive treatment. Arthritis Rheum 2008;59(2):291–6.
46. Salvarani C, Brown RD Jr, Huston J 3rd, et al. Treatment of primary CNS vasculitis with rituximab: case report. Neurology 2014;82(14):1287–8.

47. De Boysson H, Arquizan C, Guillevin L, et al. Rituximab for primary angiitis of the central nervous system: report of 2 patients from the French COVAC cohort and review of the literature. J Rheumatol 2013;40(12):2102–3.
48. Batthish M, Banwell B, Laughlin S, et al. Refractory primary central nervous system vasculitis of childhood: successful treatment with infliximab. J Rheumatol 2012;39(11):2227–9.
49. Salvarani C, Brown RD Jr, Calamia KT, et al. Primary central nervous system vasculitis: comparison of patients with and without cerebral amyloid angiopathy. Rheumatology (Oxford) 2008;47(11):1671–7.
50. Salvarani C, Brown RD Jr, Calamia KT, et al. Rapidly progressive primary central nervous system vasculitis. Rheumatology (Oxford) 2011;50(2):349–58.
51. Salvarani C, Brown RD Jr, Calamia KT, et al. Primary central nervous system vasculitis presenting with intracranial hemorrhage. Arthritis Rheum 2011;63(11): 3598–606.
52. Lian K, Siripurapu R, Yeung R, et al. Susac's syndrome. Can J Neurol Sci 2011; 38(2):335–7.
53. Bien CG, Granata T, Antozzi C, et al. Pathogenesis, diagnosis and treatment of Rasmussen encephalitis: a European consensus statement. Brain 2005; 128(Pt 3):454–71.
54. Scott RM, Smith ER. Moyamoya disease and moyamoya syndrome. N Engl J Med 2009;360:1226–37.

Kawasaki Disease

Robert P. Sundel, MD

KEYWORDS

- Vasculitis • Kawasaki disease • Coronary artery aneurysm
- Intravenous immunoglobulin • Vascular inflammation

KEY POINTS

- Many of the differences between adult and pediatric vasculitis are highlighted in Kawasaki disease, a relatively common condition in children yet essentially unknown in adults.
- Kawasaki disease is an acute, self-limited vasculitis that affects 0.01% of children during or shortly after one of many common viral and bacterial infections.
- Therapy with IVIG within 10 days of onset effectively controls the signs and symptoms of mucocutaneous inflammation and cervical lymphadenopathy characteristic of KD.
- Coronary artery inflammation with aneurysm formation is the major morbidity associated with KD; it may lead to death in >1% of untreated cases.
- IVIG prevents aneurysms more than 95% of the time, though identifying those most at risk and effectively treating resistant cases remains a challenge.

INTRODUCTION

Vasculitis means something different to a pediatrician than it does to an internist. In children, the most common forms of vasculitis, Henoch-Schönlein purpura (HSP) and Kawasaki disease (KD), have a combined incidence of almost 1/4000 (**Table 1**). These are conditions that are typically cared for by generalists, and in most cases, they resolve completely and without sequelae, if clearly delineated guidelines are followed.

The types of pediatric vasculitis that reach a rheumatologist are different. Whether the condition involves small, medium, or large vessels, these forms of vasculitis tend to be progressive and life threatening. They are largely incurable, and therefore are likely to affect pediatric patients for decades. As a result, even minor errors in treatment can lead to a widening ripple of damage and disability, which affect the rest of the child's life.

Disclosure: nothing to disclose.
Boston Children's Hospital, Rheumatology Program, 300 Longwood Avenue, and Harvard Medical School, Department of Pediatrics, 25 Shattuck Street, Boston, MA 02115, USA
E-mail address: robert.sundel@childrens.harvard.edu

Rheum Dis Clin N Am 41 (2015) 63–73
http://dx.doi.org/10.1016/j.rdc.2014.09.010
0889-857X/15/$ – see front matter © 2015 Elsevier Inc. All rights reserved.

Table 1			
KD as a reactive vasculopathy			
Feature	HSP	PAN	KD
Gender/Incidence	66% male 13.5/100,000	50% male 1/100,000	65% male 10/100,000
Trigger	33% streptococcal	30% streptococcal	~ 40% evidence of an infection
Genetic modifiers	MEFV, IgA	MEFV	CCR5, IL-4
Outcome	1% renal failure	50% systemic vasculitis	20% coronary artery lesions
Therapy	Support, steroids	Steroids, cytotoxics	95% IVIG, ~5% salvage

Abbreviations: CCR5, C-C chemokine receptor type 5; IL-4 – interleukin 4; MEFV, Mediterranean fever.

Bridging this chasm between the common and the rare is a major challenge for all clinicians, but perhaps most dramatic in the case of pediatric vasculitides. Thus, in this article various types of vascular inflammation in children are discussed: primary and secondary, self-limited and chronic, acutely life threatening and spontaneously remitting. The major focus is on key points in the natural history of the conditions at which interventions can be most effective.

EPIDEMIOLOGY

Vasculitis is rare in children. Its incidence is between 10 and 50/100,000 in various studies and populations, although all such estimates are affected by referral patterns and selection bias.[1,2] Vasculitis generally makes up less than 5% of referrals to pediatric rheumatologists, whereas if the 2 most common types, KD and HSP, are removed, they represent less than 1% of chronic inflammatory disorders of childhood.

The epidemiology of vasculitis in children sheds some light on their possible pathogenesis and in particular suggests a close connection with transmissible agents. About one-third of cases of HSP and of cutaneous polyarteritis nodosa (PAN) occur after a streptococcal infection, whereas cases of isolated angiitis of the central nervous system (CNS) often follow a viral illness.[3] A similar percentage of children with KD have evidence of an infection, although in this condition, it is concurrent with the acute manifestations of the vasculitis and may be bacterial or viral, systemic or focal.[4] Further supporting the theory that many pediatric vasculitides are triggered by transmissible agents is the fact that boys are 50% more likely than girls to develop HSP, KD, granulomatosis with polyangiitis, and PAN. The 2 most common adult vasculitides, on the other hand, giant cell arteritis and temporal arteritis, occur predominantly in women. At all ages, women's immune systems have a higher set point than men, making them more susceptible to diseases of overactive immunity and less susceptible to infections.[5]

Further epidemiologic evidence that KD is etiologically related to infections includes the fact that the average age of children with KD is about 2 years, and occurrence beyond late childhood is rare.[6] This finding suggests that the trigger is an agent or agents to which most people are exposed and become immune by late childhood. Epidemics occurred regularly in the 1980s, and during these outbreaks, the average age of patients decreased, whereas the percentage of girls increased, again typical of infections.[7] Nonetheless, decades of attempts to prove that certain viruses (eg, Epstein-Barr virus [EBV], parvovirus, human immunodeficiency virus 2), bacterial toxins (eg, streptococcal erythrogenic toxin, staphylococcal toxic shock toxin), or specific pathogens account for most cases have not been substantiated.[8] With each failure to confirm a putative agent as the cause of KD, and in view of the similarity between KD and known reactive vasculitides such as HSP and acute rheumatic fever, the greater the likelihood that KD represents a final common pathway of immune-mediated vascular inflammation after a variety of inciting infections.[9]

RISK FACTORS

Because the causes of most types of vasculitis are not known, it is not surprising that risk factors for their development are equally hidden. As noted earlier, a sizable number of cases of pediatric vasculitis follow infections or immunizations, but the overall percentage of children who develop vasculitis after exposure to these agents is vanishingly small. Genetic factors offer an attractive explanation for individual susceptibility, but even the many immunomodulatory, haplotypic, and vascular genes associated with specific vasculitides do not explain the phenomenon. Even in KD, the most thoroughly analyzed pediatric vasculitis, the relative risk conferred by polymorphisms represents only a small percentage of the overall risk of contracting the disease.[10] Only in rare cases of monogenic diseases, such as the recently identified vasculopathy associated with mutations in adenosine deaminase 2, can genetic factors reliably predict development of vasculitis. It seems that in most cases, interactions between numerous stochastic events are more important than effects of single genes, and although techniques for evaluating these factors are evolving rapidly, they are inadequate to pinpoint the cause of KD.

PATHOPHYSIOLOGY

Despite extensive research, mechanisms underlying the onset and perpetuation of vascular inflammation are poorly understood. Some aspects of the development of KD are apparently unique, whereas others likely represent stereotypical expressions of disease limited by the anatomic, physiologic, and genetic characteristics of human beings. Epidemiologic and basic studies, animal models, and response to specific biological response modifiers are shedding light on the processes involved, in particular highlighting the following.

Pathologic Characteristics

The primary target of inflammation in KD is medium-sized muscular arteries. Although a variety of nonparenchymal vessels are involved, the coronary arteries are the most severely affected, and the most likely to suffer chronic damage. Early in the process, neutrophils invade the vessel walls, and a neutrophilic infiltrate is evident in the arterial wall of fatalities that occur within the first 2 weeks of disease.[11] This process is followed by eosinophils and T cells (particularly CD8 T cells), confirmed by the presence of CD8 T cells in the arterial wall of fatalities that occur more than 2 weeks after disease onset.[12]

Immunologic Response

Gene expression studies using DNA microarrays from acute-phase KD peripheral whole blood confirmed the increased relative abundance of transcripts associated with neutrophils and acute inflammation, including adrenomedullin, grancalcin, and granulin, and decreased abundance of transcripts associated with natural killer cells and CD8+ lymphocytes.[13] In addition, the later phase of inflammation involves plasma cells (particularly IgA-producing), or macrophages, a pattern that is unique to KD.[14] Together, these findings suggest a process initiated by an innate immune response, subsequently involving a response mediated by the acquired immune system. The combination leads to rapid destruction of luminal endothelial cells, elastic lamina, and medial smooth muscle cells, with resulting loss of structural integrity, arterial wall dilatation, and aneurysm formation.

Genetic Factors

Multiple facts support a significant genetic contribution to the development of KD, mitigated by environmental factors. The incidence of the disease is significantly higher in Asian populations, lower in white populations, and intermediate among Asian families living in the United States. In one Japanese study,[15] concordance for KD was 13.3% in dizygotic twins and 14.1% in monozygotic twins, and the disease often involves succeeding generations within a single Japanese family.[16]

Many studies using differing approaches to identify candidate susceptibility loci have identified a variety of genes associated with the risk of developing KD or the severity of the disease. These genetic hotspots include histocompatibility loci as well as genes involved in vascular homeostasis and immunoregulation. No single gene explains more than 1% of a patient's risk of developing KD, so an understanding of interactions between polymorphisms is likely to be necessary before the implications of these genetic studies become evident.

Local Factors

Although coronary artery dilatation and aneurysm formation may occur in a variety of infectious (EBV), inflammatory (systemic lupus erythematosus) and vasculitic diseases (PAN), the specificity of this targeting is unique to KD. In general the characteristic predilection of different vasculitides for different anatomic sites remains unexplained, although it seems to depend on a variety of factors, including specificity of the triggering antigen, regional variations in cell surface receptors, and unidentified contributions of surrounding tissues.[17] This remains a tantalizing hint to the pathogenesis of KD, but one which has yet to even be formulated as a question that may be investigated.

CLINICAL FEATURES

The clinical evolution of KD differs from that of other, more chronic vasculitides. Characteristic of any type of vasculitis, early findings are nonspecific, primarily reflecting systemic inflammation (fever, malaise, fatigue, failure to thrive, increased levels of acute-phase reactants). However, unique to KD, progression mimics an infectious disease, with development of a rash, mucosal inflammation and extremity changes. In the early 1960s, when Tomasaku Kawasaki attempted to convince his colleagues that mucocutaneous lymph node syndrome was a unique entity, he had to distinguish it from viral exanthema and Stevens-Johnson syndrome.[18] The diagnostic criteria he established from clinical observation alone were able to identify a novel condition, and these same criteria continue to form the basis of diagnosing Dr Kawasaki's eponymous syndrome (**Box 1**).[19]

Diagnosis according to classic criteria requires the presence of fever lasting 5 days or more without any other explanation, combined with at least 4 of 5 manifestations of mucocutaneous inflammation. As with all clinical criteria, these guidelines are imperfect, with less than 100% sensitivity and specificity. Children who do not meet the criteria may have an incomplete or atypical form of KD. In addition, some patients who manifest 5 or 6 signs may have other conditions. For example, one study of patients referred for possible KD found that the standard clinical diagnostic criteria for

---

Box 1
Criteria for the diagnosis of KD (numbers in parentheses indicate approximate percentage of children with KD showing criterion)

Fever lasting 5 days or more (4 days if treatment with IVIG eradicates fever) plus at least 4 of the following clinical signs not explained by another disease process

1. Bilateral conjunctival injection (80%–90%)

2. Changes in the oropharyngeal mucous membranes (including ≥ 1 of the following symptoms: injected or fissured lips, strawberry tongue, injected pharynx) (80%–90%)

3. Changes in the peripheral extremities, including erythema or edema of the hands and feet (acute phase) or periungual desquamation (convalescent phase) (80%)

4. Polymorphous rash, primarily truncal; nonvesicular (>90%)

5. Cervical lymphadenopathy: anterior cervical lymph node at least 1.5 cm in diameter (50%)

Modified from Centers for Disease Control. Revised diagnostic criteria for Kawasaki disease. MMWR Morb Mortal Wkly Rep 1990;39(No. 44-13):27–8.

KD were fulfilled in 18 of 39 patients (46%) in whom other diagnoses were established.[20]

Kawasaki published his diagnostic guidelines before cardiac involvement was recognized in this disease. Thus, the criteria were never intended to identify children at risk for developing coronary artery abnormalities. At least 10% of children who develop coronary artery aneurysms never meet criteria for KD.[21] In an attempt to improve clinicians' ability to identify children at risk of developing coronary artery changes regardless of whether they meet classic criteria, an algorithm has been developed to diagnose and treat so-called incomplete KD.[22] Of 195 patients who developed coronary artery aneurysms from KD at 4 US centers between 1981 and 2006, 97% would have received intravenous immunoglobulin (IVIG) according to the American Heart Association (AHA) algorithm, 53 (27%) of whom would not have been treated using the classic diagnostic criteria. However, the number of children who are treated for incomplete KD without truly being at risk for developing aneurysms has not been studied.[23]

Fever is probably the most consistent manifestation of KD. It reflects increased levels of proinflammatory cytokines, such as tumor necrosis factor and interleukin 1, which are also believed to mediate the underlying vascular inflammation.[24] The fever is typically hectic, minimally responsive to antipyretic agents, and remains higher than 38.5°C during most of the illness. Because KD may be so pleomorphic, it should always be considered in a child with prolonged, unexplained fever, irritability, and laboratory signs of inflammation, especially in children younger than 12 months, in whom other manifestations of mucocutaneous inflammation are often lacking.[25]

Bilateral nonexudative conjunctivitis is present in as many as 90% of cases of KD. The predominantly bulbar injection typically begins within days of the onset of fever, and the eyes have a brilliant erythema, which spares the limbus. Children are also frequently photophobic, and anterior uveitis develops in as many as two-thirds of cases.[26] Slit-lamp examination may be helpful in ambiguous cases, because uveitis is seen more commonly in KD than in mimics of the vasculitis.

As KD progresses, mucositis often becomes evident. Cracked, red lips, and a strawberry tongue are characteristic; the latter is caused by sloughing of filiform papillae and denuding of the inflamed glossal tissue. Discrete oral lesions, such as vesicles or ulcers, as well as tonsillar exudate, suggest a viral or bacterial infection rather than KD.[20]

The cutaneous manifestations of KD may take many forms. The rash typically begins as perineal erythema and desquamation,[27] followed by macular, morbilliform, or targetoid lesions of the trunk and extremities. Vesicular or bullous lesions are rare. Changes in the extremities are generally the last manifestation of KD to develop. Children show an indurated edema of the dorsum of the hands and feet and a diffuse erythema of the palms and soles. The convalescent phase of KD may be characterized by sheetlike desquamation, which begins in the periungual region of the hands and feet.[28] Transverse depressions of the nail plates caused by temporary growth cessation during severe systemic illnesses, known as Beau lines, are another common but nonspecific feature of the convalescent phase of KD.[29] In addition, arthritis is seen in many children with KD. Arthritis most commonly affects the lower extremities, and is typically a small joint polyarthritis during the first week of illness, followed by a large joint pauciarthritis during convalescence. A retrospective review of 414 children in Toronto identified mention of arthritis in the medical records of 7.5% of cases of KD, although not all had been seen by rheumatologists or examined specifically for joint involvement.[30] Involved joints tended to be painful, but in most cases symptoms improved rapidly with routine treatment (IVIG and high-dose aspirin). In all cases, the arthritis of KD resolves, leaving no residual findings.

Cervical lymphadenopathy is the least consistent of the cardinal features of KD, absent in as many as 50% of children with the disease. When present, lymphadenopathy tends to involve primarily the anterior cervical nodes overlying the sternocleidomastoid muscle. Diffuse lymphadenopathy or other signs of reticuloendothelial involvement (eg, splenomegaly) should prompt a search for alternative diagnoses.

LABORATORY FINDINGS

Although no laboratory studies are included among the diagnostic criteria for KD, certain findings may help distinguish KD from mimics in ambiguous cases[20]:

- Systemic inflammation is most characteristic, manifested by increase of acute-phase reactants (eg, C-reactive protein, erythrocyte sedimentation rate, and α_1 antitrypsin), leukocytosis, and a left shift in the white blood cell count. By the second week of illness, platelet counts generally increase and may reach 1,000,000/ mm^3 in the most severe cases.
- Children with KD often present with a normocytic, normochromic anemia; hemoglobin concentrations more than 2 standard deviations less than the mean for age are noted in 50% of patients within the first 2 weeks of illness.
- The urinalysis commonly shows white blood cells on microscopic examination. The pyuria is of urethral origin and therefore is missed on urinalyses obtained by bladder tap or catheterization. In addition, the white cells are mononuclear and are not detected by dipstick tests for leukocyte esterase. Renal involvement may occur in KD but is uncommon.
- Measurement of liver enzymes often shows increased transaminase levels or mild hyperbilirubinemia caused by intrahepatic congestion. In addition, a few children develop obstructive jaundice from hydrops of the gallbladder.
- Other body fluids also reflect inflammation: cerebrospinal fluid (CSF) typically shows a mononuclear pleocytosis without hypoglycorrhachia or increase of CSF protein. A chart review of 46 children with KD found that 39% had increased CSF white cell counts; the median count was 22.5 cells with 6% neutrophils and 91.5% mononuclear cells, although cell counts as high as 320/mm^3 with up to 79% neutrophils were reported.[31] Similarly, arthrocentesis of involved joints shows 50 to 300,000 white cells/mm^3, primarily consisting of neutrophils.

DIFFERENTIAL DIAGNOSIS

KD is most commonly confused with infectious exanthema of childhood,[32] although other vasculitides and chronic inflammatory disorders as well as immunologic reactions may mimic KD as well:

- Measles, echovirus, and adenovirus may share many of the signs of mucocutaneous inflammation, but they typically have less evidence of systemic inflammation and generally lack the extremity changes seen in KD.
- Toxin-mediated illnesses, especially β-hemolytic streptococcal infection and toxic shock syndrome, lack the ocular and articular involvement typical of KD.
- Rocky Mountain spotted fever and leptospirosis are 2 additional infectious illnesses to be considered in the differential diagnosis of KD. Headache and gastrointestinal complaints typically are prominent features of these infections.
- Drug reactions such as Stevens-Johnson syndrome or serum sickness may mimic KD but with subtle differences in the ocular and mucosal manifestations.
- Mercury hypersensitivity reaction (acrodynia) shares certain clinical features with KD, including fever, rash, swelling of the palms and feet, desquamation, and photophobia. However, unless there is a convincing history of exposure to mercury, treatment of a child with possible KD should not be delayed while awaiting mercury levels, because acrodynia is rare in the developed world.
- Systemic-onset juvenile rheumatoid arthritis is marked by prominent rash, fever, and systemic inflammation and may be difficult to distinguish from KD until its chronicity and polyarthritis are evident. Rarely, coronary artery dilatation occurs in systemic-onset juvenile idiopathic arthritis, but changes are reversible once the systemic inflammation is controlled.[33]
- PAN involves medium-sized muscular arteries, including coronary arteries, similar to those affected by KD. The distribution of affected vessels is significantly different, as is the disease course and tempo. Nonetheless, early in the illness, especially in cases of KD that are resistant to routine therapy, the distinction may be difficult.

MANAGEMENT

Patients who fulfill the criteria for KD are hospitalized and treated with IVIG and aspirin. The AHA algorithm should be used to determine management of children with suspected KD who do not meet diagnostic criteria.[22] In such cases, based on the child's estimated risk of developing coronary artery aneurysms, the duration of fever, and supportive data including results of laboratory tests, slit-lamp examinations, and echocardiograms, treatment may be indicated, even when the diagnosis is uncertain but no clear alternative explanation for the clinical findings can be identified. Markers of increased risk of developing coronary artery aneurysms, including age less than 1 year, signs of severe systemic inflammation (especially marked anemia and left shift in the white blood cell count), and a consumptive coagulopathy, shift the balance toward empirical therapy.

Aspirin was the first medication used for treatment of KD, because of its antiinflammatory and antithrombotic effects.[34] Although aspirin was useful for management of fever and arthritis, it does not decrease the incidence of coronary artery aneurysms.[35] In view of the potential risks and lack of obvious benefits of aspirin, it should be withheld in the presence of any contraindications to its use, including bleeding, exposure to influenza or varicella, or a history of hypersensitivity to salicylates. When used, the initial dose should be no higher than 100 mg/kg/d. Once fever resolves, patients receive an antithrombotic dose of 3 to 5 mg/kg/d. Treatment with aspirin is continued until laboratory studies (eg, platelet count and sedimentation rate) return to normal.

Within the first decades after characterization of KD, children were treated with a variety of antibiotics, antithrombotic agents, and antiinflammatory medications in an attempt to shorten the course of fever and inflammation and to prevent development of coronary artery aneurysms. A cardioprotective effect in KD was first reported with IVIG in 1984.[36,37] IVIG offers a remarkable combination of efficacy and safety for the treatment of KD. Therapy within the first 10 days of illness reduces the incidence of coronary artery aneurysms by more than 70%. IVIG therapy also largely eliminates the development of giant coronary artery aneurysms (>8 mm in diameter), which are associated with the highest risk of morbidity and mortality, and rapidly restores disordered lipid metabolism and depressed myocardial contractility to normal.

Retreatment Versus Augmented Initial Therapy

Fever persists or returns 48 hours after the start of initial treatment with IVIG in 10% to 15% of patients. Persistent or recrudescent fever is particularly concerning, because it usually indicates ongoing vasculitis, reflecting a considerably increased risk of developing coronary artery aneurysms (12.2% vs 1.4% in 1 analysis).[38] Thus, it is important not to dismiss mild temperature increases in children with KD; it should be assumed that these increases represent incompletely controlled disease unless proved otherwise. Patients who remain febrile after the first dose of IVIG should be treated with a second dose of IVIG, 2 g/kg.[39]

A subgroup of patients with KD seems to be resistant to IVIG therapy, even after multiple doses. These patients are at greatest risk for development of coronary artery aneurysms and long-term sequelae of the disease. Therapies effective in other forms of vasculitis, such as corticosteroids, cyclosporine, or, at times, cyclophosphamide, have been used in these patients. Prospective studies have not compared these options, and evidence of improved cardiac outcomes are not convincing. Nonetheless, with duration of inflammation, as measured by fever, correlating most closely with coronary artery outcomes, it is difficult to withhold agents that are effective in other types of vasculitis from persistently febrile children with KD. The most effective approach seems to pair steroids with the initial dose of IVIG in children at increased risk of failing therapy with IVIG alone.[40] However, formulae that can predict IVIG resistance are imperfectly reliable, especially in non-Japanese populations, so the approach to persistent or recrudescent disease remains problematic.

PROGNOSIS

The most characteristic and specific manifestation of KD is cardiac involvement, and this factor drives all diagnostic and therapeutic decision making. KD is the leading cause of acquired heart disease in developed countries, with coronary artery aneurysms developing in almost one-quarter of untreated children and accounting for a mortality of more than 1% in the pre-IVIG era. As with acute rheumatic fever, tachycardia caused by myocarditis is nearly universal in children who develop involvement of other layers of the heart, including pericarditis and coronary arteritis. Clinically, myocardial involvement often leads to decreased contractility, commonly identifiable by an S3 gallop, which may become more prominent with hydration.

Frank aneurysms are unusual early in the course of disease, but lack of tapering seen on echocardiogram is typical, and coronary artery dimensions may be increased in the first 5 weeks after presentation. Other acute febrile illnesses may cause lesser degrees of coronary artery dilatation, which resolve more reliably than do changes because of KD.[41] With optimal current therapy, frank aneurysms with an internal diameter of 4 mm or greater are seen in only 1% to 2% of patients. Coronary artery dilatation of less than 8 mm generally regresses over time, whereas most smaller aneurysms fully resolve by echocardiogram. However, healing is by fibrointimal proliferation, and vascular reactivity does not return to normal, despite grossly normal appearance.[42] The long-term implications of such changes are unclear. A history of KD is treated at most centers as an independent risk factor for atherosclerosis, although no differences in morbidity or mortality are evident at 25-year follow-up of children whose coronary arteries are echocardiographically normal.[43]

CURRENT CONTROVERSIES

As with many areas of medicine, increasingly daunting controversies in the realm of KD are shown as layers of supposed knowledge are peeled away. Most simply, all clinicians would greatly appreciate biomarkers or other tools that would objectify a diagnostic process that is often frustratingly subjective and inexact. Each generation of analytical tools provides candidate tests, most recently urinary proteomic measures that seem to identify children with KD early and reliably.[44] However, more validation of this and other tools is necessary before any may be used clinically.

Despite such frustrations, current therapy for KD is remarkably effective: Cost-benefit analysis shows that IVIG is one of the most cost-effective medical therapies available, leading to tremendous short-term and long-term savings.[45] Nonetheless, for the 10% to 15% of children who fail IVIG treatment, options are plentiful but not nearly so beneficial. Some centers attempt to salvage such patients with intravenous pulsed dose methylprednisolone, others use infliximab, and yet others use combinations of these approaches. None is clearly effective, and reliable data based on randomized, controlled trials are needed to provide guidance.

On the most fundamental level, the question of what KD is requires a better answer. On the one hand, it is a clinical syndrome marked by fever and mucocutaneous inflammation, but therapy is directed at preventing coronary artery aneurysms, a feature not even included in the original diagnostic criteria. Guidelines for treating so-called atypical or incomplete KD have helped provide guidance in approaching children who are at risk of developing aneurysms even although they are lacking many of the findings characteristic of KD. However, it has become apparent that even conditions that are clearly not KD (such as some viral syndromes) may affect the coronaries, whereas most children who meet criteria for KD have no obvious damage to their coronary arteries. Should KD be regarded as a clinical syndrome? An echocardiographic diagnosis? A condition marked by immunologic activation and macrophage invasion of muscular arteries? Clearly, similar questions can be asked about many rheumatologic disorders, from acute rheumatic fever to systemic lupus erythematosus. Although answers are certainly beyond our ken at this time, one of the most rewarding aspects of rheumatology is that we do not have to be able to precisely define or understand the conditions we treat to be able help our patients.

REFERENCES

1. Gardner-Medwin JM, Dolezalova P, Cummins C, et al. Incidence of Henoch-Schönlein purpura, Kawasaki disease, and rare vasculitides in children of different ethnic origins. Lancet 2002;360(9341):1197–202.
2. Dolezalová P, Telekesová P, Nemcová D, et al. Incidence of vasculitis in children in the Czech Republic: 2-year prospective epidemiology survey. J Rheumatol 2004;31(11):2295–9.

3. Hayman M, Hendson G, Poskitt KJ, et al. Post-varicella angiopathy: report of a case with pathologic correlation. Pediatr Neurol 2001;24:387–9.

4. Benseler SM, McCrindle BW, Silverman ED, et al. Infections and Kawasaki disease: implications for coronary artery outcome. Pediatrics 2005;116(6):e760–6.

5. Oliver JE, Silman AJ. Why are women predisposed to autoimmune rheumatic diseases? Arthritis Res Ther 2009;11:252.

6. Burns JC, Glodé MP. Kawasaki syndrome. Lancet 2004;364:533.

7. Yanagawa H, Yashiro M, Nakamura Y, et al. Nationwide surveillance of Kawasaki disease in Japan, 1984 to 1993. Pediatr Infect Dis J 1995;14:69.

8. Principi N, Rigante D, Esposito S. The role of infection in Kawasaki syndrome. J Infect 2013;67(1):1–10.

9. Takahashi K, Oharaseki T, Yokouchi Y. Update on etio and immunopathogenesis of Kawasaki disease. Curr Opin Rheumatol 2014;26(1):31–6.

10. Onouchi Y. Genetics of Kawasaki disease: what we know and don't know. Circ J 2012;76(7):1581–6.

11. Naoe S, Takahashi K, Masuda H, Tanaka N. Kawasaki disease. With particular emphasis on arterial lesions. Acta Pathol Jpn 1991;41:785.

12. Brown TJ, Crawford SE, Cornwall ML, et al. CD8 T lymphocytes and macrophages infiltrate coronary artery aneurysms in acute Kawasaki disease. J Infect Dis 2001;184:940.

13. Popper SJ, Shimizu C, Shike H, et al. Gene-expression patterns reveal underlying biological processes in Kawasaki disease. Genome Biol 2007;8:R261, 0–261.12.

14. Jennette JC, Falk RJ. The role of pathology in the diagnosis of systemic vasculitis. Clin Exp Rheumatol 2007;25(1 Suppl 44):S52–6.

15. Harada F, Sada M, Kamiya T, et al. Genetic analysis of Kawasaki syndrome. Am J Hum Genet 1986;39(4):537–9.

16. Uehara R, Yashiro M, Nakamura Y, et al. Kawasaki disease in parents and children. Acta Paediatr 2003;92(6):694–7.

17. Hoffman GS, Calabrese LH. Vasculitis: determinants of disease patterns. Nat Rev Rheumatol 2014;10:454–62.

18. Burns JC, Kushner HI, Bastian JF, et al. Kawasaki disease: a brief history. Pediatrics 2000;106(2):1–8.

19. Kawasaki T. Acute febrile mucocutaneous syndrome with lymphoid involvement with specific desquamation of the fingers and toes in children. Arerugi 1967; 16:178 [in Japanese].

20. Burns JC, Mason WH, Glode MP, et al. Clinical and epidemiologic characteristics of patients referred for evaluation of possible Kawasaki disease. United States Multicenter Kawasaki Disease Study Group. J Pediatr 1991;118:680.

21. Sundel RP. Update on the treatment of Kawasaki disease in childhood. Curr Rheumatol Rep 2002;4:474.

22. Newburger JW, Takahashi M, Gerber MA, et al. Diagnosis, treatment, and long-term management of Kawasaki disease: a statement for health professionals from the Committee on Rheumatic Fever, Endocarditis, and Kawasaki Disease, Council on Cardiovascular Disease in the Young, American Heart Association. Pediatrics 2004;114:1708.

23. Yellen ES, Gauvreau K, Takahashi M, et al. Performance of 2004 American Heart Association recommendations for treatment of Kawasaki disease. Pediatrics 2010;125(2):e234–41.

24. Leung DY. The potential role of cytokine-mediated vascular endothelial activation in the pathogenesis of Kawasaki disease. Acta Paediatr Jpn 1991;33:739.

25. Joffe A, Kabani A, Jadavji T. Atypical and complicated Kawasaki disease in infants. Do we need criteria? West J Med 1995;162(4):322–7.
26. Blatt AN, Vogler L, Tychsen L. Incomplete presentations in a series of 37 children with Kawasaki disease: the role of the pediatric ophthalmologist. J Pediatr Ophthalmol Strabismus 1996;33(2):114–9.
27. Friter BS, Lucky AW. The perineal eruption of Kawasaki syndrome. Arch Dermatol 1988;124(12):1805–10.
28. Wang S, Best BM, Burns JC. Periungual desquamation in patients with Kawasaki disease. Pediatr Infect Dis J 2009;28(6):538–9.
29. Fimbres AM, Shulman ST. Kawasaki disease. Pediatr Rev 2008;29:308–16.
30. Gong GW, McCrindle BW, Ching JC, et al. Arthritis presenting during the acute phase of Kawasaki disease. J Pediatr 2006;148(6):800–5.
31. Dengler LD, Capparelli EV, Bastian JF, et al. Cerebrospinal fluid profile in patients with acute Kawasaki disease. Pediatr Infect Dis J 1998;17(6):478–81.
32. Yanagihara R, Todd JK. Acute febrile mucocutaneous lymph node syndrome. Am J Dis Child 1980;134:603.
33. Binstadt BA, Levine JC, Nigrovic PA, et al. Coronary artery dilation among patients presenting with systemic-onset juvenile idiopathic arthritis. Pediatrics 2005;116(1):e89–93.
34. Kusakawa S, Tatara K. Efficacies and risks of aspirin in the treatment of the Kawasaki disease. Prog Clin Biol Res 1987;250:401.
35. Durongpisitkul K, Gururaj VJ, Park JM, Martin CF. The prevention of coronary artery aneurysm in Kawasaki disease: a meta-analysis on the efficacy of aspirin and immunoglobulin treatment. Pediatrics 1995;96(6):1057–61.
36. Furusho K, Kamiya T, Nakano H, et al. High-dose intravenous gammaglobulin for Kawasaki disease. Lancet 1984;2:1055.
37. Newburger JW, Takahashi M, Burns JC, et al. The treatment of Kawasaki syndrome with intravenous gamma globulin. N Engl J Med 1986;315:341.
38. Beiser AS, Takahashi M, Baker AL, et al. A predictive instrument for coronary artery aneurysms in Kawasaki disease. US Multicenter Kawasaki Disease Study Group. Am J Cardiol 1998;81:1116.
39. Burns JC, Capparelli EV, Brown JA, et al. Intravenous gamma-globulin treatment and retreatment in Kawasaki disease. US/Canadian Kawasaki Syndrome Study Group. Pediatr Infect Dis J 1998;17:1144.
40. Son MB, Newburger JW. Management of Kawasaki disease: corticosteroids revisited. Pediatr Rev 2013;34(4):151–62.
41. Muniz JC, Dummer K, Gauvreau K. Coronary artery dimensions in febrile children without Kawasaki disease. Circ Cardiovasc Imaging 2013;6(2):239–44.
42. Senzaki H. Long-term outcome of Kawasaki disease. Circulation 2008;118:2763–72.
43. Nakamura Y, Aso E, Yashiro M, et al. Mortality among persons with a history of Kawasaki disease in Japan: can pediatricians safely discontinue follow-up of children with a history of the disease but without cardiac sequelae? Acta Paediatr 2005;94:429–34.
44. Kentsis A, Shulman A, Ahmed S, et al. Urine proteomics for discovery of improved diagnostic markers of Kawasaki disease. EMBO Mol Med 2013;5(2):210–20.
45. Klassen TP, Rowe PC, Gafni A. Economic evaluation of intravenous immune globulin therapy for Kawasaki syndrome. J Pediatr 1993;122(4):538–42.

Cogan and Behcet Syndromes

Ora Singer, MD, MS

KEYWORDS

- Behcet syndrome • Cogan syndrome • Large vessel vasculitis

KEY POINTS

- Cogan syndrome (CS) is a triad of inflammatory eye disease, vestibuloauditory dysfunction, and vasculitis.
- Consider the diagnosis of CS when inflammatory eye and ear disease present together.
- The hallmark of Behcet syndrome (BS) is mucocutaneous oral and genital ulcers, but BS can have heterogeneous manifestations.
- The possibility of large vessel involvement must be considered in all patients with CS and BS.
- Treatment of CS and BS is tailored to the disease manifestations and severity.

COGAN SYNDROME

Cogan syndrome (CS) is a rare autoimmune systemic disease, which is characterized by the combination of inflammatory eye disease and vestibuloauditory dysfunction, but it can have varied clinical manifestations. Some patients also develop a large vessel vasculitis.[1,2] Morgan and Baumgartner[3] first described the syndrome in 1934 in their case study of a patient with interstitial keratitis (IK) and Ménière disease. However, the disease is named after David G. Cogan, an ophthalmologist, who subsequently described 4 cases of "non-syphilitic IK and vestibuloauditory syndromes."[4] Seventy years after its initial description, we continue to have a limited understanding of this uncommon and pleomorphic syndrome. CS is a clinically challenging syndrome to diagnose and treat.

Epidemiology

Little is known of the prevalence and incidence of this rare disease. Approximately 250 cases have been described in the literature in all the large case series combined.[1,2,5,6]

Disclosure Statement: The author has no disclosures.
Division of Rheumatology, University of Michigan, 300 North Ingalls Street, Suite 7C27, Ann Arbor, MI 48109-5422, USA
E-mail address: singero@med.umich.edu

Disease onset is in early adulthood (20–30 years old).[1,2] Cases of children and older patients (>50 years old) have been reported. Men and women are affected equally. There is no racial or ethnic predilection. CS may be more prevalent within the population of patients with inflammatory bowel disease (IBD). Review of the literature shows 33 cases reported of overlap CS and IBD.[1,6–9]

Pathogenesis

The pathogenesis of CS is unknown. Little is learned from autopsy of temporal bone and histopathology of corneal tissue. Specimens show nonspecific lymphocytic and plasma cell infiltration.[10,11] There has not been a description of vasculitis seen on pathology in the eye or ear. However, most specimens described in the literature have been examined post mortem and are from patients who were treated with immunosuppressive agents, perhaps masking the true disease. In cases with systemic vasculitis, vessel wall histology shows acute and chronic inflammation.[12–14] One case showed a dense mononuclear infiltrate, with multiple microabscesses.[12] There have been no reports of giant cells or granulomatous inflammation.

There is increasing evidence to support autoimmunity in CS. Autoantibodies directed against antigens found in the inner ear have been identified in sera of patients with the syndrome.[15,16] Lunardi and colleagues[15] reported antibodies against a peptide that they called Cogan peptide, found in pooled sera from 8 patients with CS. This peptide shares sequence homology with CD148 and connexin 26, which are expressed both in the endothelial cell and in inner ear cells. Compelling evidence of a pathologic role for Cogan peptide comes from animal models. Passive transfer of antibodies to the peptide reproduced symptoms of CS in mice.

Another proposed target is heat shock protein 70 (HSP-70). Antibodies to HSP-70 have been reported in patients with autoimmune sensorineural hearing loss (SNHL).[16–18] In a study of patients with CS, 92% had anti-HSP-70 antibodies compared with only 5% of controls.[17] No definite role for these antibodies has been proved, and more research is needed to examine their pathogenic role.

Traditional rheumatologic antibodies such as antinuclear antibodies and rheumatoid factor have not been consistently found in CS. Although there are several case reports of antineutrophilic cytoplasmic antibodies (ANCA) associated with CS,[19,20] in larger series, ANCAs were found in a small percentage of patients with CS.[1,2]

Symptoms

CS is a multisystem disease, with heterogeneous presentations. The classic presentation as outlined in Cogan's original criteria is a triad of (1) nonsyphilitic IK, (2) vestibuloauditory symptoms, and (3) an interval between ophthalmologic and auditory symptoms of less than 2 years. A summary of the most common manifestations is presented in **Box 1**. The term atypical CS has been used to describe patients who present with a variation of these features. This presentation can include inflammatory ocular manifestations other than IK or a longer delay between eye and ear symptoms. Ocular and audiovestibular symptoms typically have a rapid onset. Either organ can present first, or they may present simultaneously. Ten percent to 15% of patients have vasculitis, which rarely is the initial presentation. IK, which results in inflammation of the cornea, is the most common eye disease. Symptoms include photophobia, pain, redness, tearing, and blurring of vision. The inner ear disease in CS is part of a group of immune-mediated inner ear diseases (IMIED), also known as autoimmune inner ear diseases (AIED). Deafness occurs in 30% to 50% of patients.[1,2,6] Long-term disease and repeated episodes may also result in the sequela of cochlear

---

Box 1
Manifestations of Cogan syndrome

Manifestation

Ocular

- IK
- Episcleritis
- Scleritis
- Choroiditis
- Uveitis
- Retinal vasculitis

Audiovestibular

- Sudden onset hearing loss (usually unilateral)
- Vertigo
- Dizziness
- Tinnitus
- Nausea
- Vomiting
- Ataxia
- Oscillopsia[a]

Vascular

- Aortitis
- Aortic and large arterial aneurysms
- Coronary arteritis
- Mesenteric vasculitis or thrombosis
- Glomerulonephritis

Systemic

- Fever
- Night sweats
- Fatigue
- Weight loss
- Lymphadenopathy
- Arthralgia and myalgia

[a] Oscillopsia is the illusion of an unstable visual field.

---

hydrops (swelling of the cochlea). This symptom presents in patients as fullness or a sensation of pressure and tinnitus, and it may also affect hearing. Often, the hydrops does not signify active disease or inflammation and should be treated without immunosuppressive drugs.

Systemic symptoms affect close to 50% of patients.[1,2,6] Typically, the vasculitis is large vessel in the form of aortitis; however, medium-sized and small vessel involvement has also been described.[14,20] All segments of the aorta and its branches are susceptible. This condition may present as aortic regurgitation, root dilatation, or aneurysm (**Fig. 1**).[12–14] Presentation may also be a pattern typical of Takayasu arteritis, with thrombosis of the aortic branches and upper extremity claudication.[21]

Diagnosis

The diagnosis of CS is clinical. There are no confirmatory blood or imaging tests. Recognition of this syndrome is challenging. Delay in diagnosis can lead to devastating outcomes. Consideration should be given to this diagnosis in all patients presenting with both eye and ear inflammatory symptoms. Slit lamp examination in early disease shows corneal infiltrates and vascularization. Rarely, in later stages, there are cells in the anterior chamber, keratitic precipitates, or scarring.[22] Audiometry is also nonspecific, showing SNHL of high and low frequencies, often sparing middle frequencies (**Fig. 2**).[1,2,5,6,23,24] Caloric testing can be performed by otolaryngology to test for vestibular dysfunction. In most cases, radiographic studies of the brain and ear are normal. MRI of the brain in the evaluation of patients with vestibular symptoms is important to exclude the possibility of tumor or stroke. There are reported cases of patients with CS with nonspecific enhancement of labyrinthine structures on T1-weighted MRI.[25,26] In a small series of 3 patients,[25] enhancement of the labyrinth on MRI correlated with disease activity and helped distinguish between active and inactive phases of disease. Studies of positron emission tomography scans in IMIED have shown early encouraging results.[27]

Laboratory testing may show signs of chronic inflammation: anemia, leukocytosis, thrombocytosis, increased inflammatory markers erythrocyte sedimentation rate (ESR) and C-reactive protein (CRP).[1,2,6] Laboratory tests to exclude other causes

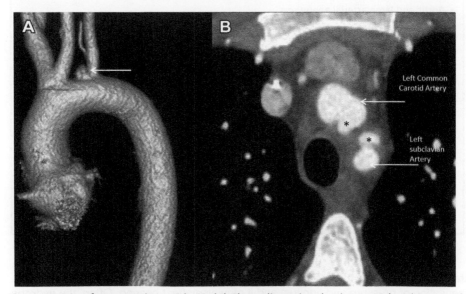

Fig. 1. Imaging from a patient with CS. (*A*) Three-dimensional volume-rendered image of the thoracic aorta from a computed tomography (CT) aortogram showing a pseudoaneurysm (*arrow*) at the origin of the left subclavian artery. (*B*) Axial contrast-enhanced CT aortogram showing concentric thickening of the aortic arch, left common carotid artery, and left subclavian artery with pseudoaneurysm (*asterisk*) formation.

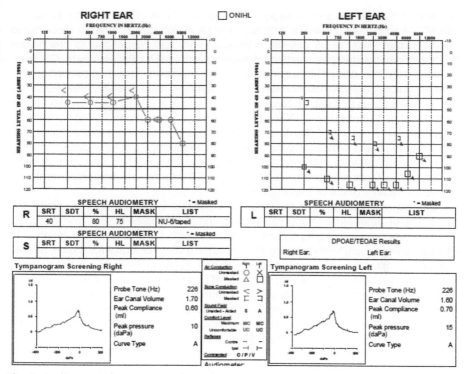

Fig. 2. Audiogram of a patient with CS showing right-ear SNHL.

should be performed, including antinuclear antibodies (ANA), extractable nuclear antigen (ENA) panel, rheumatoid factor (RF), anti-cyclic citrullinated peptide antibody (anti-CCP), ANCA, myeloperoxidase (MPO), proteinase-3 (PR3), and complements. Infectious workup may include workup for syphilis, borrelia burgdorfi, chlamydia, tuberculosis, and viruses.

Screening for vasculitis in patients with eye and ear involvement is reasonable, but there are no data to support this practice.

Management

Management and selection of treatment of CS should be tailored to the extent of disease and organ involvement. IK and other inflammatory eye diseases isolated to the anterior chambers are highly responsive to topical glucocorticoids (GC) combined with mydriatic agents. Refractory anterior disease, posterior ocular inflammatory disease, inner ear pathology, and vasculitis are indications for treatment with systemic immunosuppressive therapy.

There are no controlled trials of the treatments for SNHL and vestibular dysfunction in CS. Rapid initiation of high-dose GC has widely been accepted as the standard of care.[1,2,28–30] Prednisone 1 mg/kg/d is recommended until hearing improves, typically for 2 weeks and then tapered over 3 to 6 months. If no improvement is seen, then, a more rapid taper can be initiated. Despite good initial response, recurrent flares may lead to permanent hearing loss. There have been several open-label and retrospective studies suggesting benefit of methotrexate (MTX) as a maintenance therapy in patients with AIED and Ménière disease who had responded to high-dose steroids.[31–34] Matteson and colleagues[32] found that 11 of 17 (65%) patients treated with MTX had benefit. However, efficacy of MTX is debatable. A larger randomized controlled trial (RCT) of 65 patients with AIED who had responded to prednisone did not show greater preservation of hearing with MTX. Patients with CS were excluded from this study.[35] Other steroid-sparing therapies, including cyclophosphamide, azathioprine (AZA), leflunomide, and tacrolimus, have been reported successful in isolated cases and can be considered, but their true efficacy is unknown.[36–38] In a small trial of 23 patients with AIED, tumor necrosis factor alpha (TNFα) antagonists did not preserve hearing.[39] Rituximab was effective in improving hearing in a woman with CS with IK and vestibular symptoms.[40] Cochlear implants have been shown to be beneficial in patients with end-stage hearing loss from CS.[41,42] This surgical intervention is equally as effective in CS as in non-AIED hearing loss and significantly improves the quality of life of these patients.[42]

There are no trials to guide treatment of vasculitis in CS. Strategies parallel the paradigms of other large vessel vasculitites. Initial treatment is with high-dose GC (typically prednisone 1 mg/kg daily) for 4 weeks, with taper over 4 to 6 months. In life-threatening or organ-threatening situations, 1 g of solumedrol for 3 days as well as the concomitant use of cyclophosphamide can be considered. As has been shown in Takayasu arteritis, for more mild disease, MTX or AZA are appropriate choices.[43] Tocilizumab was shown to be effective in a man with aortitis who was unresponsive to several other immunosuppressive drugs.[44] Surgical bypass may be required for acute or chronic ischemia. However, this treatment should be reserved for scarred tissue and pursued only when disease activity is controlled.

BEHCET SYNDROME

Like CS, Behcet syndrome (BS) is a rare autoimmune systemic disease, with a hallmark clinical manifestation, in this case mucocutaenous oral ulcers, but also varied clinical manifestations. Many prefer the term Behcet syndrome to Behcet disease (BD), because of its heterogeneous presentations. It is named after Turkish physician Huluci Behcet, who in 1937 recognized the combination of oral and genital ulcers with hypopyon.[45] However, BS was likely identified many years earlier by Hippocrates, who described an endemic disease in Asia Minor characterized by "aphthous ulcerations, defluxions about the genital parts," and "watery ophthalmies."[46] The hallmark of the disease is recurrent painful oral aphthous ulcers, and most patients have genital ulcers. Symptoms can also include ophthalmologic, dermatologic, musculoskeletal, neurologic, vascular, intestinal, and pulmonary manifestations. Also like CS, BS is clinically challenging to diagnose and treat.

Epidemiology

The prevalence of BS varies by ethnic group and geographic distribution. It is most common along the ancient silk route from Asia to the Mediterranean and has its highest prevalence in Turkey (20–420/100,000).[47,48] Prevalence rates in Northern Israel are also high (15.2/100,000).[49] In comparison, the estimated prevalence rates in the United States and United Kingdom have been reported as is 5.2/100,000 and 0.64/100,000, respectively.[50] Onset is typically in young adults aged 20 to 40 years old; pediatric BS is less common.[51,52] Manifestations may also differ by region. Worldwide, men and woman are equally affected, but in the United States and Europe, the incidence is higher in women.[53] Men generally have more aggressive disease, particularly those of Middle or Far Eastern decent.[54,55]

Pathogenesis

The pathogenesis of BS is unknown. An in-depth exploration of the various mechanisms proposed is beyond the scope of this review, but a few unique pathologic features are highlighted.

BS is considered a vasculitis. Unlike other vasculitites, it affects both the venous and arterial systems and can attack vessels of all sizes. Histologic evaluation does not show classic necrotizing vasculitis, granulomas, or giant cells.[56,57] Some of the common BS lesions such as mucosal ulcers and papulopustular lesions show no vascular injury.[58] Thrombosis and arterial aneurysms (in particular, pulmonary artery aneurysm [PAA]) are also unique to BS.

The geographic distribution and familial clustering suggest a genetic predisposition to this syndrome. The strongest association has been with the HLA region and in particular HLAB51.[59] There is a significantly greater risk of developing BS in HLAB51 carriers (odds ratio 5.8). Despite these findings, HLAB51 accounts for only 20% of the disease heritability.[60] Many other non-HLA genes have been associated with BD, including genes encoding for cytokines, growth factors, and adhesion molecules. Findings by 2 independent groups of mutations in interleukin 10 (IL-10), an anti-inflammatory cytokine, are intriguing.[61,62] A recent epigenome-wide study reported aberrant DNA methylation of genes that regulate cytoskeleton dynamics, suggesting a role for epigenetics in the pathogenesis of this disease.[63]

Symptoms

BD is a multisystem disease with heterogeneous presentations. The hallmark presentation is painful aphthous oral ulcerations, which are seen in more than 95% of cases. A summary of most common manifestations is presented in **Table 1**. There are marked regional differences in disease manifestations. For example, pathergy, an abnormal skin reaction to trauma, is among the major criteria required for the diagnosis according to the International Study Group (ISG). Although pathergy occurs in 70% of Turkish cases (70%), it is rare in European and North American countries.[64] In Turkey, disease has been shown to be most severe in young men. Aggressive uveitis is common, with high rates of blindness, vascular disease, and death.[55] In contrast, a recent study from the United States showed more severe disease in women. The women affected had higher prevalence of gastrointestinal and neurologic disease. Blindness in the United States is a rare complication of uveitis in patients with BS.[50,65]

It has been proposed that symptoms of BS can present in clusters.[66] Two distinct clusters have been identified. Acne, arthritis, and enthesitis often present together and are particularly common in familial cases.[66–68] Despite the similarity to seronegative spondyloarthropathy, this subgroup is not associated with sacroileitis or HLA B27.[69] The second is a clustering of vascular manifestations. PAAs have been associated with deep venous thrombosis.[70] Furthermore, superficial and deep venous thromboses present together, as do dural sinus thrombosis and deep venous thrombosis.[71,72]

Diagnosis

Like CS, the diagnosis of BS is clinical. There are no confirmatory blood or imaging tests. Recognition of this syndrome is challenging. Delay in diagnosis can lead to devastating outcomes. Consideration should be given to this diagnosis in all patients presenting with recurrent oral and genital ulcers. Laboratory testing may show signs of chronic inflammation: anemia, leukocytosis, thrombocytosis, increase of inflammatory markers ESR and CRP.[1,2,6] Laboratory tests to exclude other causes should be

Table 1
Manifestations of BS

Manifestation	Prevalence (%)
Mucocutaneous	98
Oral ulcer	
Genital ulcers	
Dermatologic	75
Acne	
Papulopustulosis	
Erythema nodosum	
Pathergy	
Leukocytoclastic vasculitis	
Pyoderma gangrenosum	
Ocular	50–75
Uveitis	
Retinal vasculitis	
Musculoskeletal	50
Nonerosive arthritis	
Enthesitis	
Gastrointestinal	5–30
Anorexia	
Vomiting	
Diarrhea	
Central Nervous System	10–15
Parenchymal lesions	
Dural sinus thrombosis	
Intracranial hypertension	
Vascular	5–30
Superficial thrombophlebitis	
Deep venous thrombosis	
Budd-Chiari syndrome	
Arterial thrombosis	
Arterial aneurysm	
Pulmonary artery thrombosis	
Pulmonary artery aneurysm	
Cardiac	<5
Pericarditis	
Myocarditis	
Valvular disease	

performed including ANA, ENA panel, RF, anti-CCP, ANCA, MPO, PR3, and complements. Infectious workup may include workup for syphilis, Lyme, chlamydia, tuberculosis, and viruses.

There have been several classification criteria developed for BS. The most well accepted are the ISG published criteria in 1990. These criteria have been widely debated.[73] They include only the mucocutaneous, skin and eye involvement, leaving out a wide array of possible presentations. Furthermore, using these criteria, it may be difficult to distinguish BD from IBD. In 2006, the International Criteria for BD were developed in an attempt to improve the ISG criteria; vascular lesions were added, but these criteria are not widely accepted.

Management

Like in CS, management and selection of treatment of BS should be tailored to the extent of disease and organ involvement. In 2008, the European League Against Rheumatism (EULAR) published recommendations for management of BD (**Box 2**).

Mucocutaneous disease

For mild and infrequent mucosal and skin lesions, topical agents are preferred. Steroid preparations, lidocaine gel, and sucralfate suspension can be tried. Sucralfate was effective in a RCT for oral and genital ulcers.[74] Good periodontal health and oral

---

Box 2
EULAR recommendations for the management of Behcet syndrome

Any patient with BD and inflammatory eye disease affecting the posterior segment should be on a treatment regime that includes AZA and systemic corticosteroids.

If the patient has severe eye disease defined as greater than 2 lines of decrease in visual acuity on a 10/10 scale or retinal disease (retinal vasculitis or macular involvement), it is recommended that either cyclosporine A or infliximab be used in combination with AZA and corticosteroids; alternatively interferon α with or without corticosteroids could be used instead.

There is no firm evidence to guide the management of major vessel disease in BD. For the management of acute deep vein thrombosis in BD, immunosuppressive agents such as corticosteroids, AZA, cyclophosphamide, or cyclosporine A are recommended. For the management of pulmonary and peripheral arterial aneurysms, cyclophosphamide and corticosteroids are recommended.

Similarly, there are no controlled data on, or evidence of, benefit from uncontrolled experience with anticoagulants, antiplatelet, or antifibrinolytic agents in the management of deep vein thrombosis or for the use of anticoagulation for the arterial lesions of BD.

There is no evidence-based treatment that can be recommended for the management of gastrointestinal involvement of BD. Agents such as SSZ, corticosteroids, AZA, TNF-α antagonists, and thalidomide should be tried first before surgery, except in emergencies.

In most patients with BD, arthritis can be managed with colchicine.

There are no controlled data to guide the management of central nervous system involvement in BD. For parenchymal involvement, agents to be tried may include corticosteroids, interferon α, AZA, cyclophosphamide, MTX, and TNF-α antagonists. For dural sinus thrombosis, corticosteroids are recommended.

Cyclosporine A should not be used in patients with BD with central nervous system involvement unless necessary for intraocular inflammation.

The decision to treat skin and mucosa involvement depends on the perceived severity by the doctor and the patient. Mucocutaneous involvement should be treated according to the dominant or codominant lesions present.

Topical measures (ie, local corticosteroids) should be the first line of treatment of isolated oral and genital ulcers.

Acnelike lesions are usually of cosmetic concern only. Thus, topical measures as used in acne vulgaris are sufficient.

Colchicine should be preferred when the dominant lesion is erythema nodosum.

Leg ulcers in BD might have different causes. Treatment should be planned accordingly.

AZA, interferon α and TNF-α antagonists may be considered in resistant cases.

Adapted from Hatemi G, Silman A, Bang D, et al. EULAR recommendations for the management of Behcet disease. Ann Rheum Dis 2008;67(12):1656–62; with permission.

hygiene should be encouraged and are associated with lower disease activity.[75] Systemic therapy is necessary when lesions are frequent or severe and impair quality of life. Oral GC can be used for short courses to treat flares. Colchicine is the most widely used long-term steroid-sparing agent. Studies have proved it beneficial for treatment of genital ulcers and erythema nodosum, but its efficacy in addressing oral ulcers has been debated.[76–78] AZA is a good choice for resistant mucocutaneous disease.[79] Thalidomide, cyclosporine A (CSA) and interferon alpha (IFN-α) have also been studied for mucocutaneous disease and shown to be effective, but they are seldom used for this indication, because of their toxic side effect profiles.[80,81] TNF-α antagonists are usually started for other more severe indications but also treat skin and oral lesions.[82,83] Recent data on apremilast, an oral phosphodiesterase 4 inhibitor, show promise for this new drug in treatment of oral ulcers.[84] Tocilizumab, although effective for other manifestations, did not seem to work for mucocutaneous involvement.[85]

Ocular disease
The most common ocular manifestations are anterior and posterior uveitis. Eye diseases isolated to the anterior chambers are highly responsive to topical GC combined with mydriatic agents. Refractory anterior disease and posterior segment involvement mandates more aggressive therapy. Systemic GC (typically prednisone 1 mg/kg/d) is used initially to control acute inflammation with rapid taper. Steroid-sparing agents are added early in the disease course. EULAR recommends including AZA for posterior involvement. AZA reduces uveitis flares and prevents visual loss.[79,86,87] In cases of resistant disease, CSA and TNF-α antagonists should be considered. These agents can be added to AZA or patients switched to them as sole agent. CSA has the advantage of being fast acting and reduced frequency and severity of ocular attacks in several RCTs.[88–90] Several large case series support use of TNF-α antagonists in patients refractory to other disease-modifying antirheumatic drugs. Most cases have used infliximab, but there is also evidence to support the use of adalimumab and golimumab.[91–95] Etanercept is not favored. IFN-α has shown benefit in patients refractory to corticosteroids, AZA, CSA, and TNF-α antagonists.[96,97] However, its significant toxic side effect profile mandates judicious use of this drug. There are limited data to support the use of MTX or mycophenalate mofitil, and these agents should be reserved for cases in which there are no other treatment options. Reports showing efficacy of several other biologics including gevokizumab (an IL-1β antagonist), canakinumab and rituximab are encouraging, but more data is needed.[98–100]

Joint disease
The nondeforming arthritis seen in BS is usually intermittent and recurring. GC and nonsteroidal antiinflammatory drugs can be used to treat acute flares. Colchicine is generally effective. More aggressive agents, such as AZA, IFN-α, and TNF-α antagonists, although effective, are reserved for more refractory cases.

Vascular disease
Like in CS, there are no trials to guide treatment of vascular disease in BS. Strategies parallel the paradigms of other systemic vasculitides. Initial treatment is with high-dose GC. In life-threatening or organ-threatening situations, solumedrol 1 g is given for 3 days followed by a prednisone taper with concomitant use of cyclophosphamide. A retrospective case series[101] of 24 patients with PAA showed the benefit of this approach. In this series, there was high mortality despite treatment. Early data from case reports on infliximab are promising. There have been several cases of PAA

successfully treated with infliximab.[102,103] Ideally, surgery should be avoided while patients have active disease. Complication rates are high for surgical procedures, up to 24% in case series.[104] Graft occlusions and anastomotic aneurysms are most common. However, surgery is sometimes necessary for ischemic emergencies or ruptured aneurysms. Interventional radiography procedures are better tolerated and are often necessary in renal artery occlusion and peripheral arterial disease.

Thrombosis is the most common manifestation of venous disease. This complication is hypothesized to be caused by endothelial inflammation. Risk reduction for recurrent thrombus is thus best achieved with immunosuppression. AZA is the most widely used first-line agent in venous thrombosis. Anticoagulants have not been shown to be beneficial.[105] There is little data to support the use of anticoagulants. Furthermore, anticoagulation increases risks of hemorrhage in patients with aneurysms. However, indication for anticoagulation is still controversial and should be decided on a case by case basis. In critical venous disease such as central venous sinus thrombosis, Budd-Chiari syndrome, and pulmonary vein thrombosis, GC and cyclophosphamide should be considered. Infliximab was ineffective in 2 of 3 cases reported in a series of patients with BS and hepatic vein thrombosis (Budd-Chiari syndrome).[106]

Neurologic disease

There are no controlled studies to guide therapy. Parenchymal disease is treated with high-dose GC; typically solumedrol 1 g is given for 3 to 7 days (until improvement is seen), followed by a prednisone taper. For severe disease, cyclophosphamide was the steroid-sparing agent of choice, despite poor data to support its efficacy. In a small trial,[107] 4 of 7 patients with neuro-Behcet syndrome (NBS) had only a partial response to cyclophosphamide. Recent studies support use of TNF- α antagonists in NBS.[108] For milder disease, AZA is a good option to maintain disease control. CSA should be avoided in NBS. Patients treated with CSA showed worsening neurologic symptoms.[109] Tocilizumab is a promising agent. It was effective in 2 case series of patients with NBS refractory to other immunosuppressive therapies.[110,111]

Gastrointestinal disease

For mild cases of gastrointestinal involvement with BD, sulfasalazine (SSZ) or 5-amniosalicylic acid can be tried. For more severe cases, GC and AZA are first-line therapy. There are several case reports of resistant gastrointestinal symptoms responding to TNF-α antagonists (mostly infliximab). These agents can be added to SSZ or AZA. Thalidomide and INF- α have both been effective as well.

Summary

CS and BS are rare autoimmune diseases with heterogeneous manifestations. Both are considered in the spectrum of vasculitites. Because of their pleomorphic presentations, they are often missed, with delayed diagnoses and poor outcomes. Untreated disease may result in morbidity and mortality. Earlier recognition and initiation of therapy as well as the advent of new biological therapies may change the course of these syndromes.

REFERENCES

1. Haynes BF, Kaiser-Kupfer MI, Mason P, et al. Cogan's syndrome: studies in thirteen patients, long-term follow-up, and a review of the literature. Medicine 1980;59(6):426.
2. Vollertsen RS, McDonald TJ, Younge BR, et al. Cogan's syndrome: 18 cases and a review of the literature. Mayo Clin Proc 1986;61:344.

3. Morgan RF, Baumgartner CF. Meniere's disease complicated by recurrent inter-stitial keratitis: excellent results following cervical ganglionectomy. West J Surg Obstet Gynecol 1934;42:628.
4. Cogan DG. Syndrome of nonsyphilitic interstitial keratitis and vestibuloauditory syndromes. AMA Arch Ophthalmol 1945;33:144.
5. McDonald TJ, Vollertsen RS, Younge BR. Cogan's syndrome: audiovestibular involvement and prognosis in 18 patients. Laryngoscope 1985;95:650.
6. Gluth MB, Baratz KH, Matteson EL, et al. Cogan's syndrome: a retrospective review of 60 patients throughout a half century. Mayo Clin Proc 2006;81:483.
7. Froehloch F, Fried M, Gonvers JJ, et al. Association of Crohn's disease and Cogan's syndrome. Dig Dis Sci 1994;39:1134.
8. Buge A, Chamouard JM, Michin C, et al. Cogan's syndrome apropos of a case. Association with Crohn's disease. Ann Med Interne (Paris) 1986;137:75 [in French].
9. Scarl M, Frei P, Fried M, et al. Association between Cogan's syndrome and inflammatory bowel disease a case series. J Crohns Colitis 2011;5:64.
10. Schuknecht HF, Nadol JB Jr. Temporal bone pathology in a case of Cogan's syndrome. Laryngoscope 1994;104:1135.
11. Fischer ER, Hellstrom HR. Cogan's syndrome and systemic vascular disease. Analysis of pathologic features with reference to its relationship to thromboangii-tis obliterans. Arch Pathol 1961;72:572.
12. Gasparovic H, Djuric Z, Bosnic D, et al. Aortic root vasculitis associated with Cogan's syndrome. Ann Thorac Surg 2011;92:340.
13. Cochrane AD, Tatoulis J. Cogan's syndrome aortitis, aortic regurgitation and aortic arch vessel stenosis. Ann Thorac Surg 1991;52:1166.
14. Livingston JZ, Casale AS, Hutchins GM, et al. Coronary involvement in Cogan's syndrome. Am Heart J 1992;123:528.
15. Lunardi C, Bason C, Leandri M, et al. Autoantibodies to inner ear and endothe-lial antigens in Cogan's syndrome. Lancet 2002;360:915.
16. Harris JP, Sharp PA. Inner ear autoantibodies in patients with rapidly progress-ing sensorineural hearing loss. Laryngoscope 1990;100:516.
17. Bonaguri C, Orsoni J, Russo A, et al. Cogan's syndrome: anti-HSP70 antibodies are a serological marker in the typical form. Isr Med Assoc J 2014;16(5):285.
18. Billing PB, Keithley EM, Harris JP. Evidence linking the 68kDA antigen identified in progressive sensorineural hearing loss patient sera with heat shock protein 70. Ann Otol Rhinol Laryngol 1995;104:181.
19. Ikeda M, Okazaki H, Minota S. Cogan's syndrome with anti-neutrophilic anti-body. Ann Rheum Dis 2002;61:761.
20. Suzuki M, Arimura Y, Minoshima S, et al. A case of myeloperoxidase-specific anti-neutrophilic antibody (MPO-ANCA)-related glomerulonephritis associated with Cogan's syndrome. Nihon Jinzo Gakkai Shi 1996;38:423 [in Japanese].
21. Raza K, Karokis D, Kitas GD. Cogan's syndrome with Takayasu's arteritis. Br J Rheumatol 1998;37:369.
22. Cogan DG, Kuwabara T. Late corneal opacities in the syndrome of intersti-tial keratitis and vestibuloauditory symptoms. Acta Ophthalmol Suppl 1989;192:182.
23. Benitex JT, Arsenault MD, Licht JM, et al. Evidence of central vestibule-auditory dysfunction in atypical Cogan's syndrome: a case report. Am J Otol 1990;11:1311.
24. Migliori G, Battisti M, Pari N, et al. A shifty diagnosis: Cogan's syndrome. A case report and review of the literature. Acta Otorhinolaryngol Ital 2009;29:108.

25. Casselman JW, Majoor MH, Alber FW. MR of the inner ear in patients with Cogan's syndrome. AJNR Am J Neuroradiol 1994;15:131.
26. Helmchen C, Jager L, Buttner U, et al. Cogan's syndrome high resolution MRI indicators of activity. J Vestib Res 1998;8:155.
27. Mazlumzadeh M, Lowe VJ, Mullan BP, et al. The utility of positron emission tomography in the evaluation of autoimmune hearing loss. Otol Neurotol 2003; 24:201.
28. Grasland A, Ouchot J, Haculla E, et al. Typical and atypical Cogan's syndrome: 32 cases and a review of the literature. Rheumatology 2004;43:1007.
29. Haynes BF, Pikus A, Kaiser-Kupfer M, et al. Successful treatment of sudden hearing loss in Cogan's syndrome with corticosteroids. Arthritis Rheum 1981;24:501.
30. Mazlumzadeh M, Matteson E. Cogan's syndrome: an audiovestibular, ocular and systemic autoimmune disease. Rheum Dis Clin North Am 2007;33:855.
31. Matteson EL, Tirzaman O, Facer GW, et al. Use of methotrexate for autoimmune hearing loss. Ann Otol Rhinol Laryngol 2000;109:710.
32. Matteson EL, Faby DA, Fecer GE, et al. Open trial of methotrexate as treatment for autoimmune hearing loss. Arthritis Rheum 2001;45(2):146.
33. Sismanis A, Wise CM, Johnson GD. Methotrexate management of immune-mediated cochleovestibular disorders. Otolaryngol Head Neck Surg 1997; 116:146.
34. Kilpatrick JK, Sismanis AM, Spencer RF, et al. Low-dose oral methotrexate management of patients with bilateral Meniere's disease. Ear Nose Throat J 2000;79:82.
35. Harris JP, Weissman MH, Derebery JM, et al. Treatment of glucocorticoid responsive autoimmune inner ear disease with methotrexate: a randomized controlled trial. JAMA 2003;190:1875.
36. Xie L, Cai T, Bao L. Leflunomide for the successful management of Cogan's syndrome. Clin Rheumatol 2009;28:1453.
37. Roat MI, Thoft RA, Thompson AW, et al. Treatment of Cogan's syndrome with FK 506: a case report. Transplant Proc 1991;23:3346.
38. Allen NB, Cox CC, Cobo M, et al. Use of immunosuppressive agents in the treatment of severe ocular and vascular manifestations of Cogan's syndrome. Am J Med 1990;88:296.
39. Matteson EL, Choi HK, Poe DS, et al. Etanercept therapy for immune mediated cochleovestibular disorder: a multi-center, open-label pilot study. Arthritis Rheum 2005;53(3):337.
40. Orsoni JG, Lagana B, Rubino P, et al. Rituximab ameliorated severe hearing loss in Cogan's syndrome: a case report. Orphanet J Rare Dis 2010;5:18.
41. Kontorinis G, Giorgas A, Neuburger J, et al. Long-term evaluation of cochlear implantation Cogan's syndrome. ORL J Otorhinolaryngol Relat Spec 2010;72:275.
42. Wang JR, Yuen HW, Shipp DB, et al. Cochlear implantation in patients with auto-immune inner ear disease including Cogan's syndrome: a comparison with age-and sex-matched controls. Laryngoscope 2010;120:2478.
43. Unizony S, Stone JH, Stone JR. New treatment strategies for large vessel vasculitis. Curr Opin Rheumatol 2013;25:3.
44. Shibuya M, Fujio K, Morita K, et al. Successful treatment with tocilizumab in a case of Cogan's syndrome complicated with aortitis. Mod Rheumatol 2013; 23(3):577.
45. Behçet H. Über rezidiverende, apthöse durch ein Virus verursachte Geschwüre am Mund, am Auge und an der Genitalen. Dermatol Wochenschr 1937;105: 1152 [in German].

46. Feigenbaum A. Description of Behçet's syndrome in the Hippocratic third book of endemic diseases. Br J Ophthalmol 1956;40:355.
47. Azizleril G, Kose AA, Sarica R, et al. Prevalence of Behcet's disease in Istanbul, Turkey. Int J Dermatol 2003;42(10):803.
48. Yurdakul S, Gunaydin I, Tuzun Y, et al. The prevalence of Behcet's syndrome in a rural area in Northern Turkey. J Rheumatol 1988;29:1689.
49. Krause I, Yankevich A, Fraser A, et al. Prevalence and clinical aspects of Behcet's disease in the north of Israel. Clin Rheumatol 2007;26:555.
50. Calamia KT, Wilson FC, Icen M, et al. Epidemiology and clinical characteristics of Behcet's disease in the US: a population based study. Arthritis Rheum 2009; 61(5):600.
51. Tugal-Tutkun I, Urganciolu M. Childhood onset uveitis in Behcet's disease: a descriptive study of 36 cases. Am J Ophthalmol 2003;136:1114.
52. Karin-Caoglu Y, Borly M, Toker SC, et al. Demographic and clinical properties of juvenile onset Behcet's disease: a controlled multicenter study. J Am Acad Dermatol 2008;58:579.
53. Yazici Y, Moses N. Clinical manifestations and ethnic backgrounds of patients with Behcet's syndrome in US cohort. Arthrits Rheum 2007;56:S502.
54. Yazici H, Basaran G, Hamuryudan V, et al. The ten-year mortality in Behcet's syndrome. Br J Rheumatol 1996;35:139.
55. Kural-Seyahi E, Fresko I, Seyahi N, et al. The long-term morbidity and mortality of Behcet's syndrome: a 2 decade outcome survey of 387 patients followed at a dedicated medical center. Medicine 2003;82:60.
56. Meligoku M, Kural-Seyahi E, Tascilar K, et al. The unique features of vasculitis in Behcet's syndrome. Clin Rev Allergy Immunol 2008;35:40.
57. Kobayashi M, Ito M, Nakagawa A, et al. Neutrophil and endothelial cell activation in the vasa vasorum in vasculo-Behçet disease. Histopathology 2000;36:362.
58. Inoue C, Itoh R, Kawa Y, et al. Pathogenesis of mucocutaneous lesions in Behçet's disease. J Dermatol 1994;21(7):474.
59. de Menthon M, Lavalley MP, Maldini C, et al. HLA-B51/B5 and the risk of Behcet's disease: a systematic review and meta-analysis of case control genetic association studies. Arthritis Rheum 2009;61:1287.
60. Gull A, Hajeer AH, Worthington J, et al. Evidence for linkage of the HLA-B locus in Behcet's disease, obtained using the transmission disequilibrium test. Arthritis Rheum 2001;44:239.
61. Remmers EF, Cosan F, Kirino T, et al. Genome wide association study identifies variants in the MHC class I, IL10 and IL23R-IL12RB2 regions associated with Behcet's disease. Nat Genet 2010;42:698.
62. Mizuki N, Meguro A, Ota M, et al. Genome wide associations studies identify IL23R-IL12RB2 and IL10 as Behcet's disease susceptibility loci. Nat Genet 2010;42:703.
63. Hughes T, Ture-Ozdemir F, Alibaz-Oner F, et al. Epigenome-wide scan identifies a treatment-responsive pattern of altered DNA methylation among cytoskeletal remodeling genes in monocytes and CD4+ T cells from patients with Behcet's disease. Arthritis Rheum 2014;66:1648.
64. Tuzun Y, Yazici H, Pazarli H, et al. The usefulness of nonspecific skin hyper-reactivity (the pathergy test) in Behcet's in Turkey. Acta Derm Venereol 1979; 59:77.
65. Sibley C, Yazici Y, Tascilar K, et al. Behcet syndrome manifestations and activity in the Unites States versus Turkey–a cross sectional cohort comparison. J Rheumatol 2014;41:1379.

66. Diri E, Mat C, Hamuryudan V, et al. Papulopustular skin lesions are seen more frequently in patients with Behcet's syndrome who have arthritis: a controlled and masked study. Ann Rheum Dis 2001;60:1074.
67. Hatemi G, Bahar H, Uysal S, et al. Increased enthesopathy among Behcet's syndrome patients with acne and arthritis: an ultrasonography study. Arthritis Rheum 2008;58:1539.
68. Karaca M, Hatemi G, Sut N, et al. The papulopustular lesion/arthritis cluster of Behcet's syndrome also clusters in families. Rheumatology 2012;51:1053.
69. Hatemi G, Fresko I, Yurdakul S, et al. Reply to letter by Priori, et al. commenting on whether Behcet's syndrome patients with acne and arthritis compromise a true subset. Arthritis Rheum 2010;62:305.
70. Seyahi E, Melikoglu M, Akman C, et al. Pulmonary artery involvement and associated lung disease in Behcet's disease: a series of 47 patients. Medicine 2012;91:35.
71. Krause I, Leibovici L, Guedj D, et al. Disease patterns of patients with Behcet's disease demonstrated by factor analysis. Clin Exp Rheumatol 1999;17:347.
72. Tunc R, Saip S, Siva A, et al. Cerebral venous thrombosis is associated with major vessel disease in Behcet's syndrome. Ann Rheum Dis 2004;63:1693.
73. Criteria for diagnosis of Behcet's disease. International Study Group for Behcet's disease. Lancet 1990;335:1078.
74. Alpsoy E, Er H, Durusoy C, et al. The use of sucrasulfate suspension in the treatment of oral and genital ulceration of Behcet's disease: a randomized placebo-controlled double-blind study. Arch Dermatol 1999;135:529.
75. Mumcu G, Ergun T, Inanac N, et al. Oral health is impaired in Behcet's disease and is associated with disease severity. Rheumatology 2004;43:1028.
76. Aktulga E, Altac M, Muftuoglu A, et al. A double blind study of colchicine in Behcet's disease. Haematologica 1980;65:399.
77. Yurdakul S, Mat C, Tuzun Y, et al. A double blind trial of colchicine in Behcet's syndrome. Arthritis Rheum 2001;44:2686.
78. Davatchi F, Sadeghi Abdollahi B, Tehrani Banihashemi A, et al. Colchicine versus placebo in Behcet's disease: randomized double-blind, controlled crossover trial. Mod Rheumatol 2009;19:542.
79. Yazici H, Pazarli H, Barnes CG, et al. A controlled trial of azathioprine in Behcet's syndrome. N Engl J Med 1990;322:281.
80. Alpsoy E, Durusoy C, Yilmaz E, et al. Interferon alpha-2a in treatment of Behcet's disease: a randomized placebo-controlled and double blind study. Arch Dermatol 2002;138:467.
81. Hamuryudan V, Mat C, Yilmaz E, et al. Thalidomide in treatment of mucocutaneous lesions of the Behcet's syndrome: a randomized, double-blind, placebo-controlled trial. Ann Intern Med 1998;128:443.
82. Melikoglu M, Fresko I, Mat C, et al. Short term trial of etanercept in Behcet's disease–a double blind placebo controlled study. J Rheumatol 2005;32:98.
83. Arida A, Fragiadaki K, Giacvri E, et al. Anti-TNF agents for Behcet's disease: analysis of published data on 369 patients. Semin Arthritis Rheum 2011;41:61.
84. Hatemi G, Melikoglu M, Tunc R, et al. Apremilast for the treatment of Behcet's syndrome: a phase II randomized, placebo controlled double blind study. Arthritis Rheum 2013;65(Suppl 10):S322.
85. Diamantopoulos AP, Hatemi G. Lack of efficacy of tocilizumab in mucocutaneous Behcet's syndrome: report of two cases. Rheumatology 2013;52:1923.
86. Hamuryudan V, Ozyazgan Y, Hizli N, et al. Azathioprine in Behcet's syndrome: effects on long-term prognosis. Arthritis Rheum 1997;40:769.

87. Saadoun D, Wechsler B, Terrada C, et al. Azathioprine in severe uveitis of Behcet's disease. Arthritis Care Res 2010;62:1733.
88. BenExra D, Cohen E, Chajek T, et al. Evaluation of conventional therapy versus cyclosporine A in Behcet's syndrome. Transplant Proc 1988;20:136.
89. Masuda K, Nakajima A, Urayama A, et al. Double masked trial of cyclosporine versus colchicine and long term open study of cyclosporine in Behcet's disease. Lancet 1989;1:1093.
90. Ozyazgan Y, Yudakul S, Tazici H, et al. Low dose cyclosporine A versus pulse cyclophosphamide in Behcet's syndrome: a single masked trial. Br J Ophthalmol 1992;76:241.
91. Sfikakis PP, Kaklamanis PH, Elezoglou A, et al. Infliximab for recurrent, sight-threatening ocular inflammation in Adamantiades-Behçet disease. Ann Intern Med 2004;140(5):404.
92. Cantini F, Niccoli L, Nannini C, et al. Efficacy of infliximab in refractory Behçet's disease-associated and idiopathic posterior segment uveitis: a prospective, follow-up study of 50 patients. Biologics 2012;6:5.
93. Okada AA, Goto H, Ohno S, et al, Ocular Behcet's Research Group of Japan. Multicenter study of infliximab for refractory uveoretinitis in Behcet's disease. Arch Ophthalmol 2012;130:592.
94. Bawazeer A, Raffa LH, Nizamuddin SH, et al. Clinical experience with adalimumab in the treatment of ocular Behçet disease. Ocul Immunol Inflamm 2010;18(3):226.
95. Olivieri I, Leccese P, D'Angelo S, et al. Efficacy of adalimumab in patients with Behçet's disease unsuccessfully treated with infliximab. Clin Exp Rheumatol 2011;29(4 Suppl 67):S54.
96. Kötter I, Zierhut M, Eckstein AK, et al. Human recombinant interferon alfa-2a for the treatment of Behçet's disease with sight threatening posterior or panuveitis. Br J Ophthalmol 2003;87(4):423.
97. Tugal-Tutkan I, Guney-Tefekli E, Urgancioglu M, et al. Results of interferon alpha therapy in patient with Behcet's uveitis. Graefes Arch Clin Exp Ophthalmol 2006;244:1962.
98. Davatchi F, Shams H, Rezaipoor M. Rituximab in intractable ocular lesions of Behcet's disease: randomized single-blind control study (pilot study). Int J Rheum Dis 2010;13(3):246.
99. Ugurlu S, Ucar D, Seyahi E, et al. Canakinumab in patient with juvenile Behcet's syndrome–a report of 24 cases. Br J Rheumatol 1994;33:48.
100. Gul A, Tugal-Tutkun I, Dinarello CA, et al. Interleukin 1b-regulating antibody XOMA 052 (gevokizumab) in the treatment of acute exacerbations of resistant uveitis of Behcet's disease: an open label pilot study. Ann Rheum Dis 2012;71:563.
101. Hamuryudan V, Er T, Seyahi E, et al. Pulmonary artery aneurysms in Behcet's syndrome. Am J Med 2004;117:867.
102. Adler S, Baumgartner I, Villiger PM, et al. Behcet's disease: successful treatment with infliximab in 7 patients with severe vascular manifestations. A retrospective analysis. Arthritis Care Res 2012;64:607.
103. Schreiber BE, Noor N, Juli CF, et al. Resolution of Behcet's syndrome associated pulmonary arterial aneurysms with infliximab. Semin Arthritis Rheum 2011;41:482.
104. Hosaka A, Miyata T, Shigematsu H, et al. Long-term outcome after surgical treatment for arterial lesions in Behcet's disease. J Vasc Surg 2005;42:116.
105. Desbois AC, Wechsler C, Resche-Rigon M, et al. Immunosuppressants reduce venous thrombosis relapse in Behcet's disease. Arthritis Rheum 2012;64:2653.

106. Seyahi E, Hamuyudan V, Hatemi G, et al. Infliximab in the treatment of hepatic vein thrombosis in three patients with Behcet's syndrome. Rheumatology 2007;46:1213.
107. Du LT, Fain O, Wechsler B, et al. Value of 'bolus' cyclophosphamide injections in Behcet's disease: experience of 17 cases. Presse Med 1990;19:1355.
108. Fasano A, D'Agostino M, Caldarola G, et al. Infliximab monotherapy in neuro-Behcet's disease: four year follow up in a long-standing case resistant to conventional therapies. J Neuroimmunol 2011;239:105.
109. Kotter I, Gunaydin I, Batra M, et al. CNS involvement occurs more frequently in patients with Behcet's disease under cyclosporine A than under other medications–results of a retrospective analysis of 117 cases. Clin Rheumatol 2006;25:482.
110. Shapiro LS, Farrell J, Haghigi AB. Tocilixumab treatment for neuro-Behcet's disease, the first report. Clin Neurol Neurosurg 2012;114:29.
111. Urbaniak P, Hasler P, Kretzschmar S. Refractory neuro-Behcet treated by tocilixumab–a case report. Clin Exp Rheumatol 2012;30:S73.

Cold Hard Facts of Cryoglobulinemia

Updates on Clinical Features and Treatment Advances

Daniela Ghetie, MD, Navid Mehraban, MD,
Cailin H. Sibley, MD, MHS*

KEYWORDS

- Cryoglobulinemia • Cryoglobulinemic • Vasculitis • Rituximab • HCV • Diagnosis
- Treatment

KEY POINTS

- Cryoglobulins can be grouped by the Brouet classification criteria into 3 categories based on their immunoglobulin clonality. These categories have differing clinical presentations and treatment responses.
- Skin, peripheral nerves, and kidneys are the most commonly affected organs in mixed cryoglobulinemic vasculitis.
- Treatment of cryoglobulinemic vasculitis must take into account the cause of the cryoglobulins, the mechanism of damage, and the severity of symptoms.
- Most cases of cryoglobulinemic vasculitis are caused by hepatitis C virus (HCV) and advances in the identification and treatment of HCV have led to major progress in the treatment of cryoglobulinemic vasculitis.
- Mixed cryoglobulinemic vasculitis is associated with B-cell proliferation and rituximab is highly effective in the treatment of severe cases.

INTRODUCTION

Cryoglobulins consist of proteins (primarily immunoglobulins) that precipitate at temperatures less than 37°C and resolubilize when blood is heated to more than 37°C. They develop secondary to underlying inflammatory, infectious, and malignant processes but rarely can occur without an identifiable cause (ie, essential cryoglobulinemia). Cryoglobulins cause pathologic findings through 2 principal mechanisms: hyperviscosity and immune complex deposition leading to complement fixation and

Ghetie and Mehraban are co-first authors.
Disclosures: The authors have no financial disclosures to report.
Division of Arthritis & Rheumatic Diseases, Vasculitis Center, Oregon Health & Science University, Portland, OR, USA
* Corresponding author.
E-mail address: sibleyc@ohsu.edu

Rheum Dis Clin N Am 41 (2015) 93–108
http://dx.doi.org/10.1016/j.rdc.2014.09.008
0889-857X/15/$ – see front matter © 2015 Elsevier Inc. All rights reserved.

vascular inflammation. When vasculitis is present, the disease is termed cryoglobulinemic vasculitis (CryoVas). A variety of organs can be affected, leading to complex management decisions spanning gastroenterology, hematology, infectious disease, internal medicine, nephrology, neurology, and rheumatology.

BROUET CLASSIFICATION

The Brouet classification groups cryoglobulins based on their immunoglobulin clonality into 3 broad categories.[1] Types II and III consist of a polyclonal or mixed population, so they are frequently termed mixed cryoglobulins.

Type I

Type I cryoglobulinemia consists of a pure monoclonal immunoglobin[1–3] and is almost always associated with B-cell–proliferative disorders. Immunoglobulin G (IgG) and immunoglobulin M (IgM) are the most common immunoglobulins, but immunoglobulin A has been reported. Malignancies including Waldenström macroglobulinemia and multiple myeloma are the most common associations; however, monoclonal gammopathy of unclear significance can also cause disease.[4] It is the least common of the cryoglobulinemias, accounting for 10% to 15% of cases.[5]

Type II

Type II cryoglobulinemia consists of a polyclonal IgG with a monoclonal IgM directed against the polyclonal IgG.[1–3] Because a rheumatoid factor (RF) is an antibody associated with the Fc portion of IgG, patients with type II CG typically also display the RF. It is the most common type of cryoglobulinemia and is associated with hepatitis C virus (HCV) infection in 80% to 98% of cases.[6,7] Less frequent associations include hepatitis B virus (HBV)[8,9] and human immunodeficiency virus (HIV).[10]

Type III

Type III cryoglobulinemia consists of a polyclonal IgG with a polyclonal IgM and RF directed against the polyclonal IgG.[1–3] Patients usually have a background of autoimmune diseases, including lupus or Sjögren disease; however, it can also be seen secondary to HCV and lymphoproliferative disorders.[11]

EPIDEMIOLOGY

The prevalence of CryoVas is not well known; however, it is presumed to parallel the rates of local HCV infection. CryoVas presents most commonly in middle-aged individuals and is more common in women than men, with a ratio of approximately 3:1.[12] Approximately half of all patients infected with HCV have cryoglobulinemia[13,14] but only a small percentage (5%–10%) develop vasculitis.[15] Cryoglobulins can similarly be detected in the serum of patients with HBV (15%),[16] HIV (17%),[10] or connective tissue diseases (15%–25%), including systemic lupus erythematosus[17] and Sjögren syndrome,[18] but not all patients develop vasculitis.

PATHOGENESIS

The pathogenesis of type I cryoglobulinemia differs from that of mixed CryoVas. In type I, damage occurs because of hyperviscosity from high concentrations of paraproteins, resulting in sludging and eventually vascular occlusion.[19]

In contrast, B-cell stimulation and expansion are essential to the pathogenesis of mixed CryoVas. Because HCV infection is responsible for most cases, much of the progress in understanding the pathogenesis of mixed CryoVas comes from the study of HCV infection and B-cell activation. HCV viral particles in association with immune complexes with RF activity can be found in the serum cryoprecipitate and in target organ vessel walls in patients with mixed CryoVas.[20–22] The HCV envelope directly binds CD81, which is present on B cells, and allows viral entry.[23] Polyclonal expansion of marginal zone B cells then occurs, resulting in the development of immunoglobulins with RF activity.[24] Loss of B-cell regulatory control can occur, which may in part be caused by bcl-2 translocation and overexpression. This process results in a B-cell clone that produces monoclonal antibodies and may eventually lead to malignant B-cell lymphoma transformation.[25] Aberrant T-regulatory cell activity is implicated in the development of vasculitis because lower levels are present in patients with vasculitis compared with cryoglobulinemia alone, and lower levels also correlate with disease activity.[26,27] The importance of B-cell activation is further shown by the successful treatment with rituximab (RTX) (CD20 blockade), resulting in the restoration of an appropriate immune balance with a decreased number of B cells and an increased number of T-regulatory cells.[28,29] B-cell activation is similarly important in patients with mixed CryoVas with causes other than HCV, and occurs through varied mechanisms in these cases, ultimately resulting in polyclonal B-cell expansion.

CLINICAL FEATURES

Patients with type I cryoglobulinemia present with symptoms predominantly caused by complications of hyperviscosity,[4] whereas patients with mixed CryoVas display manifestations related to vasculitic involvement of organs, with hyperviscosity observed only rarely. In mixed CryoVas, skin, kidneys, and peripheral nerves are most commonly involved.[30] One of the earliest reports of cryoglobulinemic vasculitis describes a constellation of symptoms including purpura, arthralgia, and fatigue/weakness known as the Meltzer triad.[31] Subsequent studies report a broad prevalence range of 25%[11] to 80%[12] for this triad at initial presentation.

Dermatologic

Purpuric macules and papules on the lower extremities are present in almost all patients with symptomatic cryoglobulinemia.[32] In type I cryoglobulinemia, additional dermatologic manifestations at diagnosis may include acrocyanosis (30%), skin necrosis (28%), skin ulcers (27%), livedo reticularis (13%), and cold urticaria (5%).[4] Infarction and ulcers occur with lower frequency in mixed CryoVas; however, these findings are more suggestive of type I (**Fig. 1**).

Musculoskeletal

Musculoskeletal pain is a frequent manifestation, with arthralgia reported in approximately 72% of patients with mixed CryoVas.[33] This condition is typically arthralgia without frank arthritis and is not associated with florid synovitis or erosions.[30] The most common presentation is symmetric, polyarticular involvement of metacarpophalangeal joints, shoulders, knees, and ankles, which can mimic rheumatoid arthritis.[34] Arthralgia is less common in type I but is still present in 28% of patients.[4]

Renal

Renal manifestations range from isolated hematuria or proteinuria to life-threatening glomerulonephritis and acute kidney injury. Kidney disease is more prevalent in mixed CryoVas, in which it is estimated to occur in 20% to 40% of patients.[35–37]

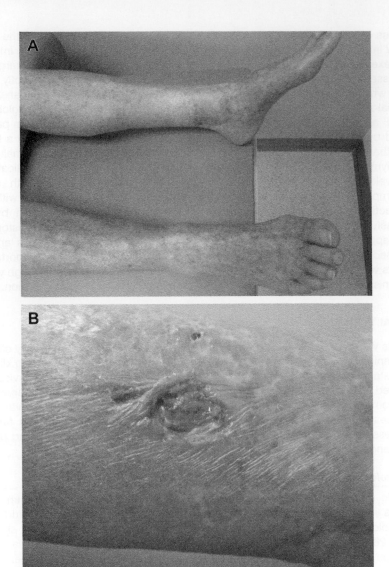

Fig. 1. Dermatologic manifestations of cryoglobulinemic vasculitis. (*A*) Palpable purpura over the lower extremity of a patient with mixed CryoVas. Hyperpigmentation at previous sites of active inflammation can be observed. (*B*) Vasculitic ulcer with surrounding purpuric macules and papules. This finding is more typical of type 1 cryoglobulinemia.

The presence of kidney disease is associated with a worse prognosis and increased mortality risk.[38]

Neurologic

Peripheral neuropathy is present in most patients with mixed cryoglobulinemia and is more prevalent in older age. The most common finding is distal symmetric sensori-motor polyneuropathy, although patients may also develop an asymmetric peripheral neuropathy, mononeuropathy, or mononeuritis multiplex.[39,40] Although approximately half of patients have evidence of neuropathy on physical examination, neuropathic findings can be detected in up to 80% of patients with the help of electrophysiologic studies.[41] The central nervous system is rarely involved; however, when this occurs, it typically manifests with cognitive impairment and white matter lesions on MRI.[42]

Pulmonary

Small airway disease and interstitial lung disease characterized by reduced expiratory flows and diffusing capacity of the lungs for carbon monoxide have been reported in patients with mixed cryoglobulinemia, but this is not a common finding.[43,44] Alveolar hemorrhage can occur with mixed CryoVas but is rare (3%) and, when present, is usually associated with kidney failure and portends a poor prognosis.[45]

Hyperviscosity

Complications related to hyperviscosity are found in patients with type I cryoglobulinemia and occur only rarely in mixed CryoVas.[12] Symptoms related to hyperviscosity include headaches, confusion, transient ischemic attacks, chest pain or heart failure, blurry vision, and oronasal bleeding.[46] Measurement of serum viscosity can be helpful in these cases because values greater than 4.0 centipoise (cp) are typically associated with clinical symptoms, whereas symptoms are rarely to never seen at values less than 3.0 cp.[47]

Other Findings

Fatigue and malaise are common in all patients. Abdominal pain is reported in a minority of patients with mixed CryoVas (7%) and may be associated with mesenteric vasculitis; however, it is not associated with worse survival.[48]

LABORATORY TESTS

The presence of cryoglobulins is essential for diagnosing cryoglobulinemic vasculitis.[49] It is critical for blood samples to be collected, stored, and centrifuged at 37°C. Improper collection and processing of samples is a frequent cause of false-negative results, particularly in centers that are inexperienced with testing. Serum is then refrigerated at 4°C for 72 hours (preferably 7 days) to promote cryoprecipitation.[50] The type of cryoglobulin (I, II, or III) is subsequently identified by electrophoresis and immunofixation. Mixed cryoglobulinemia usually generates concentrations of 1 to 5 mg/dL, whereas type I cryoglobulinemia produces much higher levels of cryoglobulins, in the range of 5 to 10 mg/dL.

Low C4 but normal to mildly diminished C3 levels are often seen in mixed cryoglobulinemia. It is not clear whether low complement levels reflect ongoing consumption or reduced synthesis because levels do not correlate with disease activity.[51] RF is detected in two-thirds of patients, with more than half of them having levels of 3 to 4 times the upper normal limit of normal; however, patients typically have a negative anti-CCP antibody.[52]

Other nonspecific features of chronic inflammatory processes that can be observed include an increased erythrocyte sedimentation rate (ESR), increased C-reactive protein level, and mild normochromic normocytic anemia. ESR can be markedly increased in type I cryoglobulinemia because of the presence of large concentrations of paraproteins.

PATHOLOGY

Type I cryoglobulinemia is characterized by noninflammatory thrombosis on biopsy of skin, kidney, or nerves. In contrast, small vessel to medium vessel vasculitis is the most common finding in patients with mixed CryoVas. A biopsy of palpable purpura reveals leukocytoclastic vasculitis.[53] In the setting of a peripheral neuropathy, a sural nerve biopsy reveals endoneural vasculitis with vessel wall destruction and with patchy, focal loss of myelinated fibers with axonal degeneneration.[54–56] Intravascular deposition of cryoglobulins in the vaso nervorum microcirculation without frank vasculitis can be seen in milder distal neuropathies.[39] When kidneys are involved, a biopsy typically shows membranoproliferative glomerulonephritis with deposition of immunoglobulin and complements in the subendothelium.[57,58] However, other histologic patterns have been reported, including focal and proliferative glomerulonephritis, membranous glomerulonephritis, and thrombotic microangiography.[35,36,59] Electron microscopy reveals glomerular dense deposits with tubular, annular, or fibrillar structures.[60]

DIAGNOSIS

A major limitation to the study and treatment of cryoglobulinemic vasculitis has been the lack of standardized classification criteria. New criteria were recently proposed by a panel of European experts from the GISC (Italian Study Group on Cryoglobulinemia)[49] and later validated in a separate large multicenter study with a sensitivity and specificity of 89.9% and 93.5%, respectively.[61] An important feature of these criteria is that cryoglobulins must be present on 2 separate occasions measured 12 weeks apart. In addition to the presence of cryoglobulins, patients must meet a set of questionnaire, clinical, and laboratory features (**Box 1**). It remains to be determined whether

---

Box 1
GISC (Italian Study Group on Cryoglobulinemia) preliminary classification criteria for cryoglobulinemic vasculitis

Must meet 2 of the following 3 items in addition to the presence of serum cryoglobulins on 2 separate occasions at least 12 weeks apart:

1. Patient questionnaire: at least 2 of the following:

   • Do you remember 1 or more episodes of small red spots on your skin, particularly involving the lower limbs?

   • Have you ever had red spots on your lower extremities that leave a brownish color after their disappearance?

   • Has a doctor ever told you that you have viral hepatitis?

2. Clinical: at least 3 of the following (past or present):

   • Constitutional symptoms: fatigue, low-grade fever 39°C to 37.9°C for more than 10 days without a cause, fever greater than 39°C without a cause, or fibromyalgia

   • Articular involvement: arthralgia or arthritis

   • Vascular involvement: purpura, skin ulcers, necrotizing vasculitis, hyperviscosity syndrome, or Raynaud phenomenon

   • Neurologic involvement

3. Laboratory: at least 2 of the following (present):

   • Reduced serum C4

   • Positive serum RF

   • Positive serum M component[49]

Adapted from De Vita S, Soldano F, Isola M, et al. Preliminary classification criteria for the cryoglobulinaemic vasculitis. Ann Rheum Dis 2011;70(7):1183–90.

these classification criteria will become adopted by the wider scientific community because additional efforts are underway to further refine classification criteria through the study endorsed by American College of Rheumatology/European League Against Rheumatism to develop diagnostic and classification criteria for vasculitis.[62]

Repeat cryoglobulin testing should be considered in the appropriate clinical setting with a negative cryoglobulin test given the frequent technical difficulties of this test. When diagnosing CryoVas, it is also important to screen for other associated conditions known to be associated with CryoVas, including HCV, HBV, HIV, autoimmune diseases, and malignancies. Screening for kidney, liver, and nervous system organ involvement should be undertaken.[63]

TREATMENT

Treatment should take into account the underlying disease (chronic viral infections, autoimmune diseases, or malignancy), the predominant mechanism of damage (hyperviscosity vs vasculitis), and the severity of the clinical manifestations (**Fig. 2**).[64,65] Although type I cryoglobulinemia differs from mixed CryoVas in its pathophysiology and clinical expression it also differs in its treatment response. This article focuses primarily on the management of the mixed CryoVas.

Type I Cryoglobulinemia

Data on type I cryoglobulinemic vasculitis are scarce; however, treatment is targeted at the underlying hematological malignancy using appropriate chemotherapy. In severe cases, additional therapy may include corticosteroids, cyclophosphamide, or

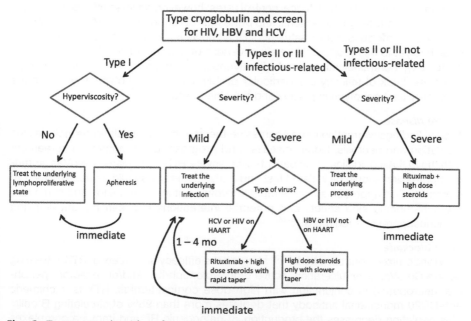

Fig. 2. Treatment algorithm for uncomplicated cryoglobulinemic vasculitis. Treatment should take into consideration the type of cryoglobulin as well as associated diseases and symptom severity. Treatment of type 1 cryoglobulinemia is directed at the underlying lymphoproliferative disease and treatment of hyperviscosity if needed. Treatment of mixed CryoVas is directed at the underlying disorder and severity of symptoms. HAART, highly active antiretroviral therapy.

biologic agents. Various regimens, including RTX, bortezomib, lenalidomide, and thalidomide, have been investigated.[66–71] All of these regimens have an efficacy rate in the range of 80%, supporting their use in naive or relapsing/refractory patients.

Mixed CryoVas

Although there are no established therapeutic protocols, the general approach to therapy in symptomatic cases includes 2 broad principles: immunosuppressive therapy and treatment of the underlying disease, with the former initiated in patients with rapidly progressive organ-threatening or life-threatening course.

Infectious Mixed CryoVas: Hepatitis C Virus Related

Mild disease

Shortly after the discovery of HCV in 1989 and its association with CryoVas, antiviral therapy became the cornerstone for management of CryoVas. In patients without severe manifestations, treatment of HCV alone, without immunosuppression, is often sufficient in achieving remission. All patients with HCV and chronic active hepatitis, except for those with decompensated cirrhosis, should receive antiviral therapy, which should be in conjunction with a hepatologist and tailored to the HCV genotype and kidney function, following the same principles as in patients with HCV infection without cryoglobulinemia. The most widely studied antiviral regimen is PEGylated interferon alfa (IFNα) and ribavirin, which results in a complete clinical response in 62.5% cases and a viral clearance of 58.3%.[72] An open-label study recently evaluated additive therapy for the protease inhibitors telaprevir or boceprevir to PEGylated IFNα and ribavirin in the treatment of HCV-associated CryoVas.[73] This treatment resulted in a higher viral clearance compared with historical control rates; however, adverse effects were common, particularly fatigue, infections, and bone marrow suppression. IFN-free regimens now exist for the successful treatment of HCV; however, their success in treating CryoVas has yet to be reported.[74] The effectiveness of current antiviral therapy is limited by toxicity, contraindications, and effectiveness in obtaining a sustained virologic response. Lack of efficacy is a particular problem in HCV genotype 1, which is the most prevalent genotype in Europe and the United States.[75,76]

Severe disease

Typical findings warranting more aggressive therapy than antivirals alone include skin ulceration and necrosis, kidney disease, and progressive neuropathy. In agreement with the EULAR guidelines,[77] in patients with severe HCV-associated CryoVas, immunosuppression should be initiated first and antiviral therapy should be delayed for 1 to 4 months. This approach achieves rapid improvement in inflammation and minimizes the confounding side effects and potential interactions between the antiviral and immunosuppressive regimens.[78–80]

CD20 blockade

Two randomized controlled trials[81,82] showed the efficacy and safety of RTX in treating severe CryoVas (skin ulceration, active glomerulonephritis, and/or refractory peripheral neuropathy) in conjunction with high-dose corticosteroids. RTX is a chimeric anti-CD20 monoclonal antibody that depletes more than 95% of circulating B cells. This depletion decreases the production of pathogenic RF and immune complexes in HCV-associated CryoVas and helps restore B-cell and T-cell immune homeostasis.[28,29]

In a multicenter randomized controlled trial, RTX (1 g intravenously [IV] at baseline and day 14 with a second dose of RTX at relapse) was compared with conventional treatment in 59 patients with severe mixed CryoVas.[81] The primary end point was survival of treatment at 12 months, which was statistically higher in the RTX group compared with conventional therapy (64.3% vs 3.5%, respectively).

A separate randomized controlled trial of RTX (375 mg/m^2/wk for 4 weeks) compared with conventional therapy was conducted in 24 patients with severe HCV-associated CryoVas in whom antiviral therapy had failed to induce remission.[82] The primary end point was clinical remission at 6 months, rather than survival of therapy. At the study end point, 83% of patients in the RTX group were in remission as measured by a Birmingham Vasculitis Activity Score (BVAS) of 0, compared with 8% of patients in the conventional therapy group (P<.001). HCV RNA levels were not affected by RTX therapy.

Because 2 separate dosing regimens have been successfully studied, there is no consensus on the choice of dosing: 4 weekly infusions of 375 mg/m^2 versus 2 biweekly infusions of 1000 mg. The lower starting dose of the weekly regimen has a theoretic advantage given the reported risk of serum sickness from increased cryoprecipitation of complexes formed by RTX with cryoglobulins.[83] Despite successful treatment with RTX, about a third of patients relapse in the first 12 months[76,84]; however, retreatment with RTX is effective in most cases.[81,82]

Cyclophosphamide

Because randomized controlled studies of RTX showed evidence of superiority compared with conventional therapy, which included cyclophosphamide, RTX is considered the optimal first-line immunosuppressive therapy. Cyclophosphamide can be considered in treatment-refractory patients and patients with adverse reactions to RTX. From uncontrolled reports and evidence of efficacy in other forms of vasculitis,[85] intermittent IV pulse cyclophosphamide as well as oral cyclophosphamide has been used for acute flares and rapidly progressive CryoVas, for which it is typically combined with plasma exchange. Close monitoring for worsening of viremia should be undertaken.

Corticosteroids

Corticosteroids are frequently initiated in the setting of severe manifestations given their rapid onset of action and control of inflammation. Because infection is the leading cause of death in patients with CryoVas,[38] corticosteroids should be used judiciously given that they increase this risk and may also worsen the underlying viral disease.[86] When necessary, a rapid taper is recommended. A typical regimen in conjunction with RTX includes pulse methylprednisolone 1 g IV for 3 days followed by prednisone 1 mg/kg orally. The dose should be decreased within 2 to 4 weeks to 40 mg with a further rapid taper to 0 within 3 months. With concurrent RTX use, this can be achieved in most patients.[82]

Infectious Mixed CryoVas: Non–Hepatitis C Virus Related

Mild disease

Although most data regarding antivirals have focused on the treatment of HCV, successful case reports and case series exist for the resolution of CryoVas after treatment of HBV.[87–90] Patients with HIV treated with highly active antiretroviral therapy (HAART) similarly have a lower rate of cryoglobulinemia.[10,91] When these infections are associated with CryoVas, they should be treated with the best available care in collaboration with appropriate consultants.

Severe disease

In contrast with HCV-associated mixed CryoVas, when immunosuppression therapy is necessary in HBV-associated or HIV-associated CryoVas because of severe disease, antiviral medication should be initiated before or at the time of immunosuppression because of the risk of worsening the underlying infection. RTX and cyclophosphamide should be avoided in patients with HBV infection,[92] patients with HIV infection not on HAART, or patients with chronic active hepatitis who are not receiving antiviral therapy because of the potentially life-threatening risk of worsening the underlying viral infection. In severe CryoVas in one of these settings, immunosuppression with corticosteroids is preferred. Corticosteroid taper should be slower than with concurrent RTX therapy given the lack of its steroid-sparing effect.

Noninfectious mixed CryoVas

In patients with mild disease, treatment options may include avoidance of cold temperature and antiinflammatory medications including nonsteroidal antiinflammatory drugs and colchicine. If an underlying autoimmune disease is identified, treatment should be focused on treating this disease.

A subgroup analysis of 2 clinical studies suggests that B-cell–depleting therapy with RTX is effective in treating noninfectious severe mixed CryoVas. Twenty-three patients from the French Autoimmunity and Rituximab registry diagnosed with nonviral Cryo-Vas were observed for 22.2 ± 16.7 months after receiving RTX.[93] RTX had clinical and immunologic efficacy and a steroid-sparing effect in all patients; however, 50% had a clinical relapse. The second study was a French multicenter CryoVas survey including 242 patients with nonviral cryoglobulinemic vasculitis.[94] RTX in combination with glucocorticoids had an almost 4-fold higher efficacy in achieving complete clinical, renal, and immunologic responses compared with glucocorticoids alone or cyclophosphamide plus corticosteroids. Serious infections were more common in patients treated with RTX, particularly in conjunction with high doses of corticosteroids.

OTHER TREATMENTS
Apheresis

Apheresis is effective at removing viral particles and immune complexes, and cryoprecipitating proteins. Although no randomized controlled studies exist, case reports and series suggest clinical efficacy of plasma exchange in life-threatening disease, including pulmonary hemorrhage and rapidly progressive glomerulonephritis.[95–98] Plasmapheresis is the first-line therapy in the treatment of symptomatic hyperviscosity,[99] although the evidence for this is sparse and based primarily on case series of hyperviscosity treatment in monoclonal gammopathies.[100,101]

A pilot open label study of low-dose interleukin-2 (IL-2) in patients with HCV-related CryoVas refractory to antivirals or RTX recently showed clinical improvement in 8 of 10 patients.[102] Investigators showed that IL-2 preferentially boosted T-regulatory cells without an increase of T-effector cells or HCV viremia. Confirmation on a larger scale as well as a better understanding of the IL-2 effects and safety profile is necessary before this therapy becomes clinically available.

SUMMARY

Cryoglobulins are produced through varied infectious, malignant, and autoimmune processes. Advances in understanding of the mechanisms responsible for the production of cryoglobulins and their pathologic consequences have led to major progress in the treatment of cryoglobulinemic vasculitis because pathogenesis and treatment are intricately connected. Although successful outcomes can now be expected in most patients, future efforts will be focused on improved treatment of associated diseases as well as the management of severe and refractory cases.

REFERENCES

1. Brouet JC, Clauvel JP, Danon F, et al. Biologic and clinical significance of cryo-globulins. A report of 86 cases. Am J Med 1974;57(5):775–88.
2. Shihabi ZK. Cryoglobulins: an important but neglected clinical test. Ann Clin Lab Sci 2006;36(4):395–408.
3. Vermeersch P, Gijbels K, Knockaert D, et al. Establishment of reference values for immunoglobulins in the cryoprecipitate. Clin Immunol 2008;129(2):360–4.
4. Terrier B, Karras A, Kahn JE, et al. The spectrum of type I cryoglobulinemia vasculitis: new insights based on 64 cases. Medicine (Baltimore) 2013;92(2): 61–8.
5. Morra E. Cryoglobulinemia. Hematology Am Soc Hematol Educ Program 2005;368–72.
6. Agnello V, Chung RT, Kaplan LM. A role for hepatitis C virus infection in type II cryoglobulinemia. N Engl J Med 1992;327(21):1490–5.
7. Misiani R, Bellavita P, Fenili D, et al. Hepatitis C virus infection in patients with essential mixed cryoglobulinemia. Ann Intern Med 1992;117(7):573–7.
8. Levo Y, Gorevic PD, Kassab HJ, et al. Liver involvement in the syndrome of mixed cryoglobulinemia. Ann Intern Med 1977;87(3):287–92.
9. Galli M, Monti G, Invernizzi F, et al. Hepatitis B virus-related markers in second-ary and in essential mixed cryoglobulinemias: a multicentric study of 596 cases. The Italian Group for the Study of Cryoglobulinemias (GISC). Ann Ital Med Int 1992;7(4):209–14.
10. Bonnet F, Pineau JJ, Taupin JL, et al. Prevalence of cryoglobulinemia and sero-logical markers of autoimmunity in human immunodeficiency virus infected indi-viduals: a cross-sectional study of 97 patients. J Rheumatol 2003;30(9): 2005–10.
11. Monti G, Galli M, Invernizzi F, et al. Cryoglobulinaemias: a multi-centre study of the early clinical and laboratory manifestations of primary and secondary dis-ease. GISC. Italian Group for the Study of Cryoglobulinaemias. QJM 1995; 88(2):115–26.
12. Ferri C, Sebastiani M, Giuggioli D, et al. Mixed cryoglobulinemia: demographic, clinical, and serologic features and survival in 231 patients. Semin Arthritis Rheum 2004;33(6):355–74.
13. Cicardi M, Cesana B, Del Ninno E, et al. Prevalence and risk factors for the pres-ence of serum cryoglobulins in patients with chronic hepatitis C. J Viral Hepat 2000;7(2):138–43.
14. Ramos-Casals M, Munoz S, Medina F, et al. Systemic autoimmune diseases in patients with hepatitis C virus infection: characterization of 1020 cases (The HIS-PAMEC Registry). J Rheumatol 2009;36(7):1442–8.
15. Vassilopoulos D, Calabrese LH. Hepatitis C virus infection and vasculitis: impli-cations of antiviral and immunosuppressive therapies. Arthritis Rheum 2002; 46(3):585–97.
16. Lunel F, Musset L, Cacoub P, et al. Cryoglobulinemia in chronic liver diseases: role of hepatitis C virus and liver damage. Gastroenterology 1994;106(5):1291–300.
17. Garcia-Carrasco M, Ramos-Casals M, Cervera R, et al. Cryoglobulinemia in sys-temic lupus erythematosus: prevalence and clinical characteristics in a series of 122 patients. Semin Arthritis Rheum 2001;30(5):366–73.
18. Ramos-Casals M, Cervera R, Yague J, et al. Cryoglobulinemia in primary Sjog-ren's syndrome: prevalence and clinical characteristics in a series of 115 pa-tients. Semin Arthritis Rheum 1998;28(3):200–5.

19. Della Rossa A, Tavoni A, Bombardieri S. Hyperviscosity syndrome in cryoglobulinemia: clinical aspects and therapeutic considerations. Semin Thromb Hemost 2003;29(5):473–7.

20. Sansonno D, Cornacchiulo V, Iacobelli AR, et al. Localization of hepatitis C virus antigens in liver and skin tissues of chronic hepatitis C virus-infected patients with mixed cryoglobulinemia. Hepatology 1995;21(2):305–12.

21. Sansonno D, Gesualdo L, Manno C, et al. Hepatitis C virus-related proteins in kidney tissue from hepatitis C virus-infected patients with cryoglobulinemic membranoproliferative glomerulonephritis. Hepatology 1997;25(5):1237–44.

22. Ferri S, Dal Pero F, Bortoletto G, et al. Detailed analysis of the E2-IgM complex in hepatitis C-related type II mixed cryoglobulinaemia. J Viral Hepat 2006;13(3): 166–76.

23. Pileri P, Uematsu Y, Campagnoli S, et al. Binding of hepatitis C virus to CD81. Science 1998;282(5390):938–41.

24. Rosa D, Saletti G, De Gregorio E, et al. Activation of naive B lymphocytes via CD81, a pathogenetic mechanism for hepatitis C virus-associated B lymphocyte disorders. Proc Natl Acad Sci U S A 2005;102(51):18544–9.

25. Zignego AL, Ferri C, Giannelli F, et al. Prevalence of bcl-2 rearrangement in patients with hepatitis C virus-related mixed cryoglobulinemia with or without B-cell lymphomas. Ann Intern Med 2002;137(7):571–80.

26. Boyer O, Saadoun D, Abriol J, et al. CD4+CD25+ regulatory T-cell deficiency in patients with hepatitis C-mixed cryoglobulinemia vasculitis. Blood 2004;103(9): 3428–30.

27. Landau DA, Rosenzwajg M, Saadoun D, et al. Correlation of clinical and virologic responses to antiviral treatment and regulatory T cell evolution in patients with hepatitis C virus-induced mixed cryoglobulinemia vasculitis. Arthritis Rheum 2008;58(9):2897–907.

28. Saadoun D, Rosenzwajg M, Landau D, et al. Restoration of peripheral immune homeostasis after rituximab in mixed cryoglobulinemia vasculitis. Blood 2008; 111(11):5334–41.

29. Holz LE, Yoon JC, Raghuraman S, et al. B cell homeostasis in chronic hepatitis C virus-related mixed cryoglobulinemia is maintained through naive B cell apoptosis. Hepatology 2012;56(5):1602–10.

30. Frankel AH, Singer DR, Winearls CG, et al. Type II essential mixed cryoglobulinaemia: presentation, treatment and outcome in 13 patients. QJM 1992;82(298): 101–24.

31. Meltzer M, Franklin EC. Cryoglobulinemia–a study of twenty-nine patients. I. IgG and IgM cryoglobulins and factors affecting cryoprecipitability. Am J Med 1966; 40(6):828–36.

32. Cohen SJ, Pittelkow MR, Su WP. Cutaneous manifestations of cryoglobulinemia: clinical and histopathologic study of seventy-two patients. J Am Acad Dermatol 1991;25(1 Pt 1):21–7.

33. Gorevic PD, Kassab HJ, Levo Y, et al. Mixed cryoglobulinemia: clinical aspects and long-term follow-up of 40 patients. Am J Med 1980;69(2):287–308.

34. Weinberger A, Berliner S, Pinkhas J. Articular manifestations of essential cryoglobulinemia. Semin Arthritis Rheum 1981;10(3):224–9.

35. D'Amico G. Renal involvement in hepatitis C infection: cryoglobulinemic glomerulonephritis. Kidney Int 1998;54(2):650–71.

36. Roccatello D, Fornasieri A, Giachino O, et al. Multicenter study on hepatitis C virus-related cryoglobulinemic glomerulonephritis. Am J Kidney Dis 2007; 49(1):69–82.

37. Matignon M, Cacoub P, Colombat M, et al. Clinical and morphologic spectrum of renal involvement in patients with mixed cryoglobulinemia without evidence of hepatitis C virus infection. Medicine (Baltimore) 2009;88(6):341–8.
38. Landau DA, Scerra S, Sene D, et al. Causes and predictive factors of mortality in a cohort of patients with hepatitis C virus-related cryoglobulinemic vasculitis treated with antiviral therapy. J Rheumatol 2010;37(3):615–21.
39. Garcia-Bragado F, Fernandez JM, Navarro C, et al. Peripheral neuropathy in essential mixed cryoglobulinemia. Arch Neurol 1988;45(11):1210–4.
40. Gemignani F, Pavesi G, Fiocchi A, et al. Peripheral neuropathy in essential mixed cryoglobulinaemia. J Neurol Neurosurg Psychiatry 1992;55(2):116–20.
41. Ferri C, La Civita L, Cirafisi C, et al. Peripheral neuropathy in mixed cryoglobulinemia: clinical and electrophysiologic investigations. J Rheumatol 1992;19(6):889–95.
42. Casato M, Saadoun D, Marchetti A, et al. Central nervous system involvement in hepatitis C virus cryoglobulinemia vasculitis: a multicenter case-control study using magnetic resonance imaging and neuropsychological tests. J Rheumatol 2005;32(3):484–8.
43. Bombardieri S, Paoletti P, Ferri C, et al. Lung involvement in essential mixed cryoglobulinemia. Am J Med 1979;66(5):748–56.
44. Viegi G, Fornai E, Ferri C, et al. Lung function in essential mixed cryoglobulinemia: a short-term follow-up. Clin Rheumatol 1989;8(3):331–8.
45. Amital H, Rubinow A, Naparstek Y. Alveolar hemorrhage in cryoglobulinemia–an indicator of poor prognosis. Clin Exp Rheumatol 2005;23(5):616–20.
46. Ramos-Casals M, Stone JH, Cid MC, et al. The cryoglobulinaemias. Lancet 2012;379(9813):348–60.
47. Crawford J, Cox EB, Cohen HJ. Evaluation of hyperviscosity in monoclonal gammopathies. Am J Med 1985;79(1):13–22.
48. Terrier B, Saadoun D, Sene D, et al. Presentation and outcome of gastrointestinal involvement in hepatitis C virus-related systemic vasculitis: a case-control study from a single-centre cohort of 163 patients. Gut 2010;59(12):1709–15.
49. De Vita S, Soldano F, Isola M, et al. Preliminary classification criteria for the cryoglobulinaemic vasculitis. Ann Rheum Dis 2011;70(7):1183–90.
50. Vermeersch P, Gijbels K, Marien G, et al. A critical appraisal of current practice in the detection, analysis, and reporting of cryoglobulins. Clin Chem 2008;54(1):39–43.
51. Tarantino A, Anelli A, Costantino A, et al. Serum complement pattern in essential mixed cryoglobulinaemia. Clin Exp Immunol 1978;32(1):77–85.
52. Wener MH, Hutchinson K, Morishima C, et al. Absence of antibodies to cyclic citrullinated peptide in sera of patients with hepatitis C virus infection and cryoglobulinemia. Arthritis Rheum 2004;50(7):2305–8.
53. Dupin N, Chosidow O, Lunel F, et al. Essential mixed cryoglobulinemia. A comparative study of dermatologic manifestations in patients infected or noninfected with hepatitis C virus. Arch Dermatol 1995;131(10):1124–7.
54. Nemni R, Corbo M, Fazio R, et al. Cryoglobulinaemic neuropathy. A clinical, morphological and immunocytochemical study of 8 cases. Brain 1988;111(Pt 3):541–52.
55. Tredici G, Petruccioli MG, Cavaletti G, et al. Sural nerve bioptic findings in essential cryoglobulinemic patients with and without peripheral neuropathy. Clin Neuropathol 1992;11(3):121–7.
56. Cavaletti G, Petruccioli MG, Crespi V, et al. A clinico-pathological and follow up study of 10 cases of essential type II cryoglobulinaemic neuropathy. J Neurol Neurosurg Psychiatry 1990;53(10):886–9.

57. Tarantino A, De Vecchi A, Montagnino G, et al. Renal disease in essential mixed cryoglobulinaemia. Long-term follow-up of 44 patients. QJM 1981;50(197):1–30.
58. Beddhu S, Bastacky S, Johnson JP. The clinical and morphologic spectrum of renal cryoglobulinemia. Medicine (Baltimore) 2002;81(5):398–409.
59. Herzenberg AM, Telford JJ, De Luca LG, et al. Thrombotic microangiopathy associated with cryoglobulinemic membranoproliferative glomerulonephritis and hepatitis C. Am J Kidney Dis 1998;31(3):521–6.
60. Ben-Bassat M, Boner G, Rosenfeld J, et al. The clinicopathologic features of cryoglobulinemic nephropathy. Am J Clin Pathol 1983;79(2):147–56.
61. Quartuccio L, Isola M, Corazza L, et al. Validation of the classification criteria for cryoglobulinaemic vasculitis. Rheumatology (Oxford) 2014. [Epub ahead of print].
62. Craven A, Robson J, Ponte C, et al. ACR/EULAR-endorsed study to develop Diagnostic and Classification Criteria for Vasculitis (DCVAS). Clin Exp Nephrol 2013;17(5):619–21.
63. Invernizzi F, Pietrogrande M, Sagramoso B. Classification of the cryoglobulinemic syndrome. Clin Exp Rheumatol 1995;13(Suppl 13):S123–8.
64. Retamozo S, Brito-Zeron P, Bosch X, et al. Cryoglobulinemic disease. Oncology (Williston Park) 2013;27(11):1098–105, 1110–6.
65. Perez-Alamino R, Espinoza LR. Non-infectious cryoglobulinemia vasculitis (CryoVas): update on clinical and therapeutic approach. Curr Rheumatol Rep 2014; 16(5):420.
66. Besada E, Vik A, Koldingsnes W, et al. Successful treatment with bortezomib in type-1 cryoglobulinemic vasculitis patient after rituximab failure: a case report and literature review. Int J Hematol 2013;97(6):800–3.
67. Payet J, Livartowski J, Kavian N, et al. Type I cryoglobulinemia in multiple myeloma, a rare entity: analysis of clinical and biological characteristics of seven cases and review of the literature. Leuk Lymphoma 2013;54(4):767–77.
68. Nehme-Schuster H, Korganow AS, Pasquali JL, et al. Rituximab inefficiency during type I cryoglobulinaemia. Rheumatology (Oxford) 2005;44(3):410–1.
69. Pandrangi S, Singh A, Wheeler DE, et al. Rituximab treatment for a patient with type I cryoglobulinemic glomerulonephritis. Nat Clin Pract Nephrol 2008;4(7): 393–7.
70. Calabrese C, Faiman B, Martin D, et al. Type 1 cryoglobulinemia: response to thalidomide and lenalidomide. J Clin Rheumatol 2011;17(3):145–7.
71. Lin RJ, Curran JJ, Zimmerman TM, et al. Lenalidomide for the treatment of cryoglobulinemia and undifferentiated spondyloarthropathy in a patient with multiple myeloma. J Clin Rheumatol 2010;16(2):90–1.
72. Saadoun D, Resche-Rigon M, Thibault V, et al. Antiviral therapy for hepatitis C virus–associated mixed cryoglobulinemia vasculitis: a long-term followup study. Arthritis Rheum 2006;54(11):3696–706.
73. Saadoun D, Resche Rigon M, Thibault V, et al. Peg-IFNalpha/ribavirin/protease inhibitor combination in hepatitis C virus associated mixed cryoglobulinemia vasculitis: results at week 24. Ann Rheum Dis 2014;73(5):831–7.
74. Sulkowski MS, Gardiner DF, Rodriguez-Torres M, et al. Daclatasvir plus sofosbuvir for previously treated or untreated chronic HCV infection. N Engl J Med 2014; 370(3):211–21.
75. St Clair EW. Hepatitis C virus-related cryoglobulinemic vasculitis: emerging trends in therapy. Arthritis Rheum 2012;64(3):604–8.
76. Ferri C, Cacoub P, Mazzaro C, et al. Treatment with rituximab in patients with mixed cryoglobulinemia syndrome: results of multicenter cohort study and review of the literature. Autoimmun Rev 2011;11(1):48–55.

77. Mukhtyar C, Guillevin L, Cid MC, et al. EULAR recommendations for the management of primary small and medium vessel vasculitis. Ann Rheum Dis 2009;68(3):310–7.
78. Petrarca A, Rigacci L, Caini P, et al. Safety and efficacy of rituximab in patients with hepatitis C virus-related mixed cryoglobulinemia and severe liver disease. Blood 2010;116(3):335–42.
79. Batisse D, Karmochkine M, Jacquot C, et al. Sustained exacerbation of cryoglobulinaemia-related vasculitis following treatment of hepatitis C with peginterferon alfa. Eur J Gastroenterol Hepatol 2004;16(7):701–3.
80. Lidove O, Cacoub P, Hausfater P, et al. Cryoglobulinemia and hepatitis c: worsening of peripheral neuropathy after interferon alpha treatment. Gastroenterol Clin Biol 1999;23(3):403–6 [in French].
81. De Vita S, Quartuccio L, Isola M, et al. A randomized controlled trial of rituximab for the treatment of severe cryoglobulinemic vasculitis. Arthritis Rheum 2012; 64(3):843–53.
82. Sneller MC, Hu Z, Langford CA. A randomized controlled trial of rituximab following failure of antiviral therapy for hepatitis C virus-associated cryoglobulinemic vasculitis. Arthritis Rheum 2012;64(3):835–42.
83. Sene D, Ghillani-Dalbin P, Amoura Z, et al. Rituximab may form a complex with IgMkappa mixed cryoglobulin and induce severe systemic reactions in patients with hepatitis C virus-induced vasculitis. Arthritis Rheum 2009;60(12):3848–55.
84. Cacoub P, Delluc A, Saadoun D, et al. Anti-CD20 monoclonal antibody (rituximab) treatment for cryoglobulinemic vasculitis: where do we stand? Ann Rheum Dis 2008;67(3):283–7.
85. Houwert DA, Hene RJ, Struyvenberg A, et al. Effect of plasmapheresis (PP), corticosteroids and cyclophosphamide in essential mixed polyclonal cryoglobulinaemia associated with glomerulonephritis. Proc Eur Dial Transplant Assoc 1980;17:650–4.
86. Ciesek S, Steinmann E, Iken M, et al. Glucocorticosteroids increase cell entry by hepatitis C virus. Gastroenterology 2010;138(5):1875–84.
87. Cakir N, Pamuk ON, Umit H, et al. Successful treatment with adefovir of one patient whose cryoglobulinemic vasculitis relapsed under lamivudine therapy and who was diagnosed to have HBV virologic breakthrough with YMDD mutations. Intern Med 2006;45(21):1213–5.
88. Enomoto M, Nakanishi T, Ishii M, et al. Entecavir to treat hepatitis B-associated cryoglobulinemic vasculitis. Ann Intern Med 2008;149(12):912–3.
89. Stecevic V, Pevzner MM, Gordon SC. Successful treatment of hepatitis B-associated vasculitis with lamivudine. J Clin Gastroenterol 2003;36(5):451.
90. Boglione L, D'Avolio A, Cariti G, et al. Telbivudine in the treatment of hepatitis B-associated cryoglobulinemia. J Clin Virol 2013;56(2):167–9.
91. Kosmas N, Kontos A, Panayiotakopoulos G, et al. Decreased prevalence of mixed cryoglobulinemia in the HAART era among HIV-positive, HCV-negative patients. J Med Virol 2006;78(10):1257–61.
92. Mitka M. FDA: increased HBV reactivation risk with ofatumumab or rituximab. JAMA 2013;310(16):1664.
93. Terrier B, Launay D, Kaplanski G, et al. Safety and efficacy of rituximab in nonviral cryoglobulinemia vasculitis: data from the French Autoimmunity and Rituximab registry. Arthritis Care Res 2010;62(12):1787–95.
94. Terrier B, Krastinova E, Marie I, et al. Management of noninfectious mixed cryoglobulinemia vasculitis: data from 242 cases included in the CryoVas survey. Blood 2012;119(25):5996–6004.

95. Rockx MA, Clark WF. Plasma exchange for treating cryoglobulinemia: a descriptive analysis. Transfus Apher Sci 2010;42(3):247–51.
96. Madore F, Lazarus JM, Brady HR. Therapeutic plasma exchange in renal diseases. J Am Soc Nephrol 1996;7(3):367–86.
97. Guillevin L, Pagnoux C. Indications of plasma exchanges for systemic vasculitides. Ther Apher Dial 2003;7(2):155–60.
98. Campise M, Tarantino A. Glomerulonephritis in mixed cryoglobulinaemia: what treatment? Nephrol Dial Transplant 1999;14(2):281–3.
99. Szczepiorkowski ZM, Winters JL, Bandarenko N, et al. Guidelines on the use of therapeutic apheresis in clinical practice–evidence-based approach from the Apheresis Applications Committee of the American Society for Apheresis. J Clin Apher 2010;25(3):83–177.
100. Reinhart WH, Lutolf O, Nydegger UR, et al. Plasmapheresis for hyperviscosity syndrome in macroglobulinemia Waldenstrom and multiple myeloma: influence on blood rheology and the microcirculation. J Lab Clin Med 1992;119(1):69–76.
101. Menke MN, Feke GT, McMeel JW, et al. Effect of plasmapheresis on hyperviscosity-related retinopathy and retinal hemodynamics in patients with Waldenstrom's macroglobulinemia. Invest Ophthalmol Vis Sci 2008;49(3): 1157–60.
102. Saadoun D, Rosenzwajg M, Joly F, et al. Regulatory T-cell responses to low-dose interleukin-2 in HCV-induced vasculitis. N Engl J Med 2011;365(22): 2067–77.

Vasculitis in Antiphospholipid Syndrome

Lindsay Lally, MD*, Lisa R. Sammaritano, MD

KEYWORDS

- Antiphospholipid syndrome • Vasculitis • Lupus anticoagulant
- Anticardiolipin antibody • Anti-β2-glycoprotein 1 antibody

KEY POINTS

- Systemic vasculitis may rarely coexist with antiphospholipid syndrome (APS), despite the fact that the classic APS manifestations are thrombosis and vasculopathy.
- Vasculitic-like manifestations attributed to antiphospholipid antibodies (aPL) include livedoid vasculitis, retinal vasculitis, and diffuse alveolar hemorrhage.
- Antiphospholipid antibodies are increased in certain primary vasculitic disorders; a causative association of aPL with thrombosis in these patients has not been shown, however, and routine testing for aPL in primary vasculitis is not recommended.
- Differentiating between vasculitis and antiphospholipid-associated thrombosis, especially in patients with known primary vasculitis or systemic lupus, is critical in determining appropriate immunosuppressive or anticoagulant therapy.

INTRODUCTION

Antiphospholipid syndrome (APS) is an autoimmune disease characterized by vascular thrombosis and/or pregnancy morbidity occurring in conjunction with serologically detectable antiphospholipid antibodies (aPL). aPL, defined as autoantibodies directed against phospholipid-binding plasma proteins, include lupus anticoagulant (LAC), anticardiolipin antibody (aCL), and anti–β2-glycoprotein I (aβ2GPI), and should be persistently positive when measured at least 12 weeks apart to meet the criteria for APS (**Box 1**).[1] Detection of positive aPL in the absence of characteristic clinical events does not equate to a diagnosis of APS; many individuals with positive aPL remain asymptomatic indefinitely. Because transient aPL positivity can be triggered by certain infections, malignancies, or medications, demonstration of persistent serologic

Disclosure Statement: The authors have nothing to disclose.
Division of Rheumatology, Hospital for Special Surgery, 535 East 70th Street, New York, NY 10021, USA
* Corresponding author.
E-mail address: lallyl@hss.edu

> **Box 1**
> **Updated classification criteria for definite antiphospholipid syndrome (APS)**
>
> *Clinical Criteria*
>
> 1. Vascular thrombosis:
>
>   At least 1 clinical episode of arterial, venous, or small vessel thrombosis, in any tissue or organ
>
> 2. Pregnancy morbidity:
>
>   a. At least 1 unexplained death of a morphologically normal fetus at or beyond the 10th week of gestation, or
>
>   b. At least 1 premature birth of a morphologically normal neonate before the 34th week of gestation because of eclampsia, severe preeclampsia, or recognized features of placental insufficiency, or
>
>   c. At least 3 unexplained consecutive spontaneous abortions before the 10th week of gestation, with maternal anatomic or hormonal abnormalities, and paternal and maternal chromosomal causes excluded
>
> *Laboratory Criteria[a]*
>
> 1. Lupus anticoagulant present in plasma
>
> 2. Anticardiolipin antibody of immunoglobulin (Ig)G and/or IgM isotype, in medium or high titer (>40 IgG or IgM phospholipid units)
>
> 3. Anti–β2-glycoprotein I antibody of IgG and/or IgM isotype in medium or high titer (>99th percentile)
>
> Definite APS is present if at least 1 of the clinical and 1 of the laboratory criteria are met.
> [a] Laboratory criteria must be present on 2 or more occasions at least 12 weeks apart.

positivity is critical when considering a diagnosis of APS. APS may occur alone or in the setting of another autoimmune disease, most commonly systemic lupus erythematosus (SLE).

Although venous or arterial thrombosis and fetal loss are the commonest clinical manifestations of APS, this is a multisystem disease with many noncriteria manifestations including thrombocytopenia, skin ulcers, nephropathy, and cardiac valvular disease.[2] The pathogenic vascular lesions in APS are predominantly related to thrombosis or microangiopathy and not inflammation. However, vascular inflammation, namely, vasculitis, may rarely be a component of APS.[3] Furthermore, aPL positivity or secondary APS may occur in patients with an underlying primary systemic vasculitis.[4,5]

ANTIPHOSPHOLIPID ANTIBODIES, ANTIPHOSPHOLIPID SYNDROME, AND VASCULITIS

The mechanistic interplay between aPL and vascular inflammation is complex. Although the pathogenesis of thrombosis in APS is not entirely understood, the interactions of aPL with antigenic components of the phospholipid complex are essential in mediating the pathologic prothrombotic phenotype.[6] Subsequent endothelial cell activation and damage contributes to the vasculopathy of APS.

Despite the persistent presence of aPL, clinically evident thrombosis occurs only occasionally, suggesting that a "second hit" is required for the development of thrombosis. Inflammation driven by the nuclear factor κB pathway and/or complement activation has been hypothesized as a link between the aPL-induced hypercoagulable state and frank thrombus development.[7] Endothelial cell activation, production of inflammatory cytokines, and upregulation of vascular adhesion molecules promote the recruitment of neutrophils and monocytes to the vascular lumen.[6,7] Thus, an inflammatory cell infiltrate may coexist with thrombosis in APS; however, this is a reactive process and does not represent true vasculitis with the pathognomonic inflammation of the vessel wall.

When histopathologic vasculitis is found in APS, it is usually a contemporaneous phenomenon and is not causally related to the APS.[8] Concurrent vasculitis and APS most commonly occur in a patient with SLE or another underlying connective tissue disease.[9] Vasculitis occurs in approximately 10% to 35% of SLE patients, with small-vessel cutaneous vasculitis accounting for 80% of cases; aPL antibodies are found in 40% of SLE patients.[10–12] Albeit infrequently, SLE patients can develop medium-vessel or large-vessel vasculitis that affects the central or peripheral nervous system or visceral organs. In characterizing vasculitis in large cohorts of SLE patients, a correlation between vasculitis, aPL, and APS-related manifestations such as livedo reticularis, venous thrombosis, and thrombocytopenia has been reported.[10,12] Despite the association between vasculitis and aPL in SLE, however, there is no evidence to support a causative role of aPL in the development of vasculitis.[4,13]

The link between aPL positivity and SLE vasculitis may relate to damage of the vascular endothelium by the vasculitic process.[10,14] Disruption of the vascular endothelium exposes phospholipids that, together with phospholipid-binding proteins, can serve as an antigenic stimulus for aPL production and/or a binding target for circulating aPL. This same mechanism of vasculitic damage may also explain the association of aPL and APS with primary systemic vasculitis. Prevalence estimates of definite APS occurring in the primary systemic vasculitides range from 0.7% to 6%, although the prevalence of aPL positivity in these conditions is much higher.[5,15] APL have been reported in association with all of the primary systemic vasculitides, including those affecting small, medium, and large vessels.

The sequelae of vascular occlusion, whether thrombotic or inflammatory, are tissue ischemia and end-organ damage, and can be clinically indistinguishable. There is an obvious need to differentiate between thrombotic and vasculitic lesions to guide therapy and choose between anticoagulation and immunosuppression. The remainder of this article focuses first on a discussion of the reported vasculitic manifestations of APS itself, then on the significance of aPL in the individual vasculitic syndromes.

VASCULITIC MANIFESTATIONS OF ANTIPHOSPHOLIPID SYNDROME
Cutaneous Lesions

A variety of dermatologic manifestations have been described in APS.[16] Cutaneous lesions occur in approximately half of patients with APS, with livedo reticularis being the most frequent dermatologic manifestation.[17] Livedoid vasculitis, also known as livedo reticularis with ulceration, has been described in APS and is characterized by purpuric lesions of the lower extremities that progress to ulceration and atrophie blanche (**Fig. 1**).[18] Despite the name, the histopathology of livedoid vasculitis lacks evidence of true vasculitis, without perivascular inflammatory infiltrate or leukocytoclasia, and is more properly termed livedoid vasculopathy. Patients with APS can also present with painful cutaneous nodules resembling cutaneous vasculitis. However, these lesions are typically refractory to immunosuppression and demonstrate thrombosis of superficial dermal vessels on biopsy without vasculitis; thus, these nodules are termed pseudovasculitis.[17,19,20] There have been several reports of APS patients with histopathologic leukocytoclastic vasculitis on biopsy, but most of these patients had concurrent SLE.[17,21] In a small cohort of patients with underlying connective

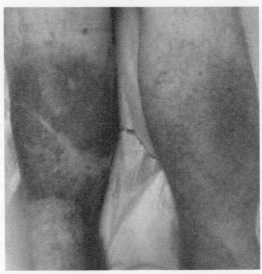

Fig. 1. Livedoid "vasculitis" with atrophie blanche in a patient with antiphospholipid syndrome. (*Courtesy of* Michael Lockshin, MD, Hospital for Special Surgery, New York.)

tissue disease, immunoglobulin (Ig)A but not IgG aCL positivity was associated with cutaneous vasculitic lesions in 9 patients who did not have any other manifestations of APS.[22]

Retinal Vasculitis

Ocular manifestations are not uncommon in APS[23]; most of these are caused by occlusive ocular vascular disease, which may also be associated with central nervous system involvement.[24] Frank retinal vasculitis, with or without concurrent retinal thrombosis, can occur in APS.[25,26] In a cohort of patients presenting with ocular inflammatory disease who were found to have aCL positivity, retinal vasculitis was diagnosed in 60% of aCL-positive patients.[27] However, only 3 of the 13 patients with retinal vasculitis in this cohort had high-titer aCL IgG (>40) and repeat aCL testing was not available, making the diagnosis of definite APS difficult to establish.

A diagnosis of retinal vasculitis is made on the basis of characteristic fluorescein angiographic findings of vascular leakage and capillary nonperfusion. Thus, retinal vasculitis in APS is not based on histopathologic evidence, so the presence of microthrombi as the underlying etiologic trigger cannot be excluded. The cases of reported retinal vasculitis in APS were all treated successfully with anticoagulation without immunosuppression, further supporting a thrombotic etiology.[25,26]

Diffuse Alveolar Hemorrhage

Diffuse alveolar hemorrhage (DAH), disruption of the alveolar-capillary basement membrane resulting in bleeding into the alveolar space, is a rare but serious manifestation of APS.[28] DAH occurs more frequently in the catastrophic antiphospholipid syndrome (CAPS) than in classic APS.[29] Presentation of DAH can vary from dyspnea and cough to hemoptysis and acute respiratory failure. The histopathologic lesion of DAH in APS/CAPS is pulmonary capillaritis, which is believed to be immune mediated. In the largest reported series of primary APS-associated DAH, 18 patients were described; histologic evidence of capillaritis was noted in all 3 patients who underwent surgical lung biopsy.[30] Bronchial alveolar lavage demonstrates neutrophilia, and neutrophils are often present in the alveolar space on biopsy specimens even if capillaritis is not seen.[31] These inflammatory pathologic findings in APS-associated DAH occur in the absence of thrombosis; thus, DAH is considered to be a nonthrombotic manifestation of APS.

The pathogenic mechanism leading to capillary damage or capillaritis in APS-associated DAH is not well understood. Circulating aPL are believed to be pathogenic in this inflammatory manifestation of APS[32] and may induce upregulation of endothelial cell-adhesion molecules, with ensuing neutrophil recruitment and migration into the alveolar space and resultant tissue destruction and hemorrhage.[30,31]

The presumed inflammatory nature of DAH in APS has important therapeutic implications. Experts recommend prompt initial treatment of DAH with high-dose corticosteroids and temporary cessation of anticoagulation.[28,30] Additional immunosuppression is often needed, as recurrences and mortality are common. No controlled or prospective data are available to guide treatment of APS-related DAH; however, borrowing from the treatment of capillaritis in antineutrophil cytoplasmic antibody (ANCA)-associated vasculitis, cyclophosphamide (CYC) or rituximab (RTX) are often the first-line agents used. In a recent retrospective series from the Mayo Clinic of 18 patients with primary APS-associated DAH, complete remission was achieved in 3 of 7 patients treated with CYC and 5 of 8 patients treated with an RTX-based regimen, whereas uncontrolled disease was observed in patients treated with azathioprine, mycophenolate mofetil, intravenous Ig, or plasmapheresis.[30]

Miscellaneous Case Reports

Biopsy-proven vasculitis in association with primary APS has been reported in a variety of organ systems (**Table 1**). There are case reports of cerebral vasculitis,

Table 1
Vasculitic manifestations reported in primary antiphospholipid syndrome (APS)

Organ System	Clinical Manifestation	Histopathology	Comments
Skin	Livedoid vasculitis, pseudovasculitis	Fibrinoid changes, fibrin plugs along vascular channels, thrombi in superficial dermal vessels	Despite term livedoid vasculitis, this is believed to be a thrombotic vasculopathy
Ocular	Retinal vasculitis	No abnormality, diagnosed on basis of fluorescein angiography	May be related to microthrombosis in retinal vasculature
Pulmonary	Diffuse alveolar hemorrhage	Capillaritis and/or neutrophilia in alveolar space	Considered to be a nonthrombotic manifestation of APS
Cardiac[a]	Myocardial infarction	Coronary arteritis and thrombosis	
Renal[a]	Hypertension	Immune-complex vasculitis reported in one case	
Central nervous system[a]	Stroke, encephalopathy	Granulomatous angiitis	
Peripheral nervous system[a]	Mononeuritis multiplex	Necrotizing arteritis with thrombosis	

[a] Case reports only.

diagnosed on brain biopsy, in patients with persistent LAC positivity and no signs of underlying SLE.[33,34] These patients were uniformly treated with high-dose corticosteroids, although 1 of the 3 reported cases proved fatal despite immunosuppression. Vasculitic involvement of peripheral nerves has also been reported in a woman with aCL and recurrent pregnancy loss who developed mononeuritis multiplex with sural nerve biopsy confirming vasculitis.[35] Arteritis in the coronary arteries with concurrent thrombosis was identified in the autopsy of a woman with LAC and aCL positivity and recurrent venous thromboembolism who suffered a fatal myocardial infarction.[36] Occlusive involvement of the renal artery resulting from vasculitis presenting as hypertension has also been reported in primary APS.[37,38]

ANTIPHOSPHOLIPID ANTIBODIES AND ANTIPHOSPHOLIPID SYNDROME IN SYSTEMIC VASCULITIS

The systemic vasculitides are a heterogeneous group of disorders characterized by the common feature of vascular inflammation. The 2012 revised Chapel Hill Consensus Conference provides a useful classification for the primary vasculitides based chiefly on the caliber of the vessels involved in the inflammatory process.[39] Although aPL have been reported in conjunction with all of the systemic vasculitides, the pathogenic significance of these autoantibodies in vasculitis is under debate.

Small-Vessel Vasculitis

Antineutrophil cytoplasmic antibody–associated vasculitis
The ANCA-associated vasculitides (AAV), which include granulomatosis with polyangiitis (GPA, formerly Wegener granulomatosis), microscopic polyangiitis (MPA), and eosinophilic granulomatosis with polyangiitis (EGPA, formerly Churg-Strauss syndrome), are a group of multisystem autoimmune diseases characterized by necrotizing small- to medium-vessel vasculitis and the presence of serologically detectable ANCA. In a study of prevalence of aCL antibodies in patients with various connective tissue diseases, 3.8% of patients with AAV were aCL-positive, a prevalence paralleling the healthy control population.[40]

There are scattered case reports of APS occurring in the context of all of the subtypes of AAV.[41,42] As in APS, patients with AAV can present with pulmonary capillaritis and DAH. There are 2 reports of pulmonary capillaritis occurring in GPA patients with concurrent APS and deep venous thrombosis.[43,44] In both cases, the investigators causally attributed DAH to GPA but hypothesized that thrombosis was related to the presence of aPL interacting with damaged endothelium.

This relationship between aPL and AAV has been most extensively explored in GPA. GPA patients are at an increased risk of venous thromboembolism.[45,46] The Wegener's granulomatosis Clinical Occurrence of Thrombosis Study (WeCLOT), using a cohort of 180 GPA patients enrolled in a randomized clinical trial, calculated the incidence of venous thromboembolic events to be 7 per 100 person-years.[45] This rate was 20-fold higher than that in the general population and 7-fold higher than that observed in SLE patients. Venous thromboembolic events were temporally associated with periods of active disease.

To further explore hypercoagulability in active GPA, aCL and aβ2GPI antibody titers in the WeCLOT cohort were ascertained.[47] Although aCL were found in 12% of the GPA patients, almost all were IgM isotype and there were no high-titer antibodies. Five patients (3%) had aβ2GPI positivity; again, these antibodies were low titer and predominantly IgM. There were no differences in aPL positivity between patients who had experienced a venous thromboembolic event and those who had not; thus, presence of aPL cannot explain the high incidence of venous thromboembolism in GPA. A 10% to 25% prevalence of aPL positivity that does not correlate with thrombosis has been corroborated in other GPA cohorts.[14,48] APL in GPA are generally low titer, sometimes with resolution of aPL positivity on repeat testing.[47,49,50] In addition, other noncriteria APS manifestations such as thrombocytopenia are not associated with the presence of aPL in GPA patients.[51] One series of 5 patients with GPA and EGPA, positive aPL, and uncontrolled hypertension reported renal artery stenosis in the absence of atheromata: the investigators speculated that the renal artery stenosis may have been partial thromboses related to aPL.[52]

A related condition whereby ANCA and aPL coexist is the cutaneous vasculopathy associated with levamisole-adulterated cocaine use. Levamisole, an anthelminthic agent used as a cocaine additive, has been implicated as the pathogenic antigen in the development of a vasculitic syndrome that includes neutropenia, retiform purpura with cutaneous necrosis, and autoantibody production. Approximately 90% of patients with levamisole-induced vasculopathy have a detectable ANCA, usually perinuclear ANCAs directed against atypical antigens such as human neutrophil elastase.[53] LAC and aCL are also frequently detected in this syndrome; a review of 61 patients with levamisole-associated vasculopathy noted LAC positivity in 50% and IgM aCL positivity in 65% of patients.[54] Biopsy of the cutaneous lesions reveals concurrent small-vessel vasculitis and thrombosis in one-third of cases, suggesting that both the ANCA and the aPL may be mechanistically important in the development of the clinical phenotype.

Though rare, medication-induced syndromes are also described: propylthiouracil and the anti–tumor necrosis factor α drug infliximab have been reported to induce concurrent aPL and vasculitis.[55,56]

Henoch-Schönlein purpura

Henoch-Schönlein purpura (HSP), or IgA vasculitis, is a small-vessel immune-complex–mediated vasculitis associated with leukocytoclasia and IgA deposition. HSP is the most common systemic vasculitis in the pediatric population, characterized by palpable purpura in conjunction with joint, gastrointestinal, or renal involvement.

Patients with acute HSP have an increased number of circulating IgA-producing cells, often with increased IgA levels during active disease.[57,58] Investigators have found aCL IgA antibodies in 75% of adults and pediatric patients with acute HSP[59–61]; levels of aCL IgA correlate with C-reactive protein and interleukin-6 levels in adult HSP, with an association between IgA aCL and renal involvement in one report.[62] However, thrombotic events were not detected in any of the patients with IgA aCL, and most patients had undetectable IgA aCL antibody titers on repeat convalescent testing. One group found an association between central nervous system involvement of HSP and aPL in the serum and cerebrospinal fluid of 46 affected children[63]; however, clinical information and details on aPL isotype and titer were not reported.

The etiology of HSP is unknown, although many experts believe there is an infectious trigger with an antigenic stimulus leading to increased IgA production.[57] Infection is also a well-known stimulus for aPL production (most commonly non-IgG isotypes); in most cases the infection-induced aPL are not pathogenic.[64] Thus, detection of IgA aPL in active HSP may be reflective of an infectious exposure, and may not have specific pathogenic or prognostic implications.

Medium-Vessel Vasculitis

Polyarteritis nodosa

Polyarteritis nodosa (PAN) is a necrotizing vasculitis of medium-sized muscular arteries, and skin, nervous system, gastrointestinal, and renal involvement are common. A focal, segmental vasculitis with fibrinoid necrosis is the characteristic pathologic lesion of PAN on biopsy. Angiographic demonstration of microaneurysms is an acceptable surrogate for histopathologic confirmation for the diagnosis of PAN.[65] Unlike AAV, patients with PAN do not seem to be at an increased risk for thromboembolic events.[66]

There are several case reports documenting coexistence of classic PAN and APS.[4,67–72] In one small cohort of 13 patients with PAN, 30% were aPL positive but no patients had an aPL-associated thrombotic event.[14] Several reports describing coexisting PAN and APS present histopathologic evidence of vasculitis, or angiographic demonstration of microaneurysms and frank thrombosis in the presence of serologically detected aPL; treatment with immunosuppression and anticoagulation were initiated simultaneously.[59,61,62] Other cases, however, were treated successfully with immunosuppression alone, with disappearance of aPL on repeat testing.[60,63] Primary APS may also present with visceral aneurysms as are seen in PAN, which further complicates the association between these 2 conditions, especially in the absence of histologic documentation of vasculitis or thrombosis.[37,73] The distinction between PAN and APS in the presence of visceral aneurysms is not trivial, as anticoagulation in the presence of aneurysms may confer increased risk of bleeding from a ruptured aneurysm: every effort should be made to confirm the diagnosis of APS in these rare cases.

One group has suggested an association of antiphosphatidylserine-prothrombin complex antibodies (aPS/PT) with a mild variant of PAN, cutaneous PAN (CPN). Elevated levels of IgG and IgM aPS/PT were identified in a series of patients with CPN without evidence of thrombosis.[74]

Large-Vessel Vasculitis

Giant-cell arteritis

Giant-cell arteritis (GCA) is a granulomatous inflammatory disorder of medium and large blood vessels affecting the aorta and its major branches that occurs in adults older than 50 years. With an annual incidence between 19 and 30 per 100,000 population, GCA is the most common systemic vasculitis in adults.[75] The most feared complication of untreated GCA is visual loss from ischemic optic neuropathy. Approximately 20% of patients with GCA will develop either unilateral or bilateral blindness, which usually occurs early in the disease course.[76]

The presence of aPL has been explored in GCA to a greater extent than any of the other systemic vasculitides. The relationship between GCA and aPL was initially described by Cid and colleagues[77] in a patient with biopsy-proven GCA, elevated IgM aCL, and arteriogram suggestive of arterial thrombosis in the bilateral lower extremities. The same group subsequently reported aCL in 3 of 40 (7.5%) patients with biopsy-positive GCA.[78] Other studies have reported higher incidences of aCL, with IgG and IgM isotypes detected in 20% to 50% of GCA patients.[79–81] By contrast, in a cohort of 45 GCA patients, no patients had aβ2GPI despite aCL positivity in half.[82] Detectable aPL have been described in patients with polymyalgia rheumatica (PMR) in association with GCA, although aPL are typically negative in patients with isolated PMR.[83]

Despite the high prevalence of aCL in GCA, there does not appear to be an association between aCL and ischemic events.[81,84] In a longitudinal study of serial aCL measurements in 58 GCA patients, aCL was initially positive in 27 patients but normalized with treatment in all but 1.[85] An increase in aCL titer was documented in 20 of 27 (74%) disease flares and paralleled an increase in acute-phase reactants. Presence of aCL had no relationship with prognosis, treatment response, or presenting signs or symptoms in GCA, and has been hypothesized to be a marker of endothelial damage. Endothelial disruption may uncover immunologically active antigens and stimulate antiendothelial antibodies, which may include aPL.[86] As such, most experts recommend against routine testing for aPL in GCA.[87]

Takayasu arteritis

Takayasu arteritis (TAK) is a granulomatous, large-vessel vasculitis predominantly affecting the aorta and its branches. Unlike GCA, TAK is generally a disease of young women, with a female to male ratio of 8.5 to 1 and most cases presenting before age 40 years.[88] The reported prevalence of aPL positivity in TAK patients is variable, ranging from 0% to 53%.[89–92] As in other vasculitides such as GCA, the presence of aPL in TAK corresponds with antiendothelial cell antibodies and disease activity.[90,92] When detected in TAK, aPL are most likely an epiphenomenon reflecting damage to the vascular endothelium; however, some investigators speculate that the presence of aPL may contribute to the obstructive vasculopathy of late TAK following the initial inflammatory phase.

There are few case reports in the literature of patients with APS presenting with large-vessel involvement in a TAK-like distribution.[93] There is debate in the literature as to the significance of aortic occlusive disease in primary APS[94,95]; whether this lesion is thrombotic or inflammatory is not readily distinguishable with conventional imaging, and tissue is rarely accessible.[96] However, in most case reports patients were successfully treated with corticosteroids, suggesting an inflammatory etiology. Use of PET imaging has been suggested as a modality to help distinguish between thrombosis and inflammation in APS with suspected large-vessel involvement.[97]

Variable-Vessel Vasculitis

Behçet syndrome

Behçet syndrome is a systemic vasculitis that can involve small, medium, or large vessels in the arterial or venous system. Recurrent oral and genital ulcers are a hallmark of Behçet syndrome. Other manifestations can include skin lesions, arthritis, uveitis, gastrointestinal ulceration, and vascular involvement. Pulmonary artery aneurysm and/or thrombosis are severe manifestations of Behçet syndrome, and carry 25% to 30% mortality.[98] Pulmonary arterial disease is also associated with peripheral vascular disease, typically presenting as thrombophlebitis with superficial or deep venous thrombosis. Thrombi in Behçet syndrome are usually surrounded by an inflammatory infiltrate.[99] Management of venous thrombosis in Behçet syndrome is controversial, but most experts support treatment with immunosuppression rather than anticoagulation.[100]

The frequency and clinical associations of aPL have been investigated in several cohorts of Behçet patients. APL were first detected in 13 of 70 Behçet patients from a mixed European and Middle Eastern cohort, with a statistically significant association between aCL and retinal vascular involvement.[101] This association with ocular disease was confirmed in a second cohort of 20 patients, with aPL detectable in 35% and associated with presence of uveitis.[102] Tokay and colleagues[103] subsequently found a much lower frequency of aPL positivity (7%) in a large cohort of Turkish patients. In a pooled analysis of 23 studies looking at aCL in more than 900 Behçet patients, the overall frequency of aCL was 19.2%. Regional variation in aCL was reported with positivity in only 9.5% of Turkish patients with Behçet syndrome compared with 25% in other populations. Importantly an association between aPL and thrombotic events has not been well established in this disorder.[104–106]

FUTURE CONSIDERATIONS AND SUMMARY

Although vasculopathy and thrombosis remain the hallmark of APS, considerable evidence suggests that APS is at least in part mediated through inflammatory immune-system mechanisms and that vasculitis may rarely represent a manifestation of this systemic autoimmune disorder. Vasculitis may be particularly significant in the noncriteria manifestation of DAH.

More commonly aPL likely coexist with vasculitis in connective tissue diseases such as SLE, whereby differentiating between inflammatory and thrombotic causes of vascular damage remains challenging. The significance of aPL in the primary vasculitides is less certain, and may represent the result of endothelial cell damage or an epiphenomenon. It is worthwhile to be alert to the possibility of concomitant APS in these disorders, however, as treatment options differ: true APS-induced thrombosis mandates anticoagulation in addition to immunosuppressive therapy.

REFERENCES

1. Miyakis S, Lockshin MD, Atsumi T, et al. International consensus statement on an update of the classification criteria for definite antiphospholipid syndrome (APS). J Thromb Haemost 2006;4:295–306.
2. Erkan D, Lockshin MD. Non-criteria manifestations of antiphospholipid syndrome. Lupus 2010;19:424–7.
3. Lie JT. Vasculopathy of the antiphospholipid syndromes revisited: thrombosis is the culprit and vasculitis the consort. Lupus 1996;5:368–71.
4. Norden DK, Ostrov BE, Shafritz AB, et al. Vasculitis associated with antiphospholipid syndrome. Semin Arthritis Rheum 1995;24:273–81.
5. Rees JD, Lanca S, Marques PV, et al. Prevalence of the antiphospholipid syndrome in primary systemic vasculitis. Ann Rheum Dis 2006;65:109–11.
6. Giannakopoulos B, Krilis SA. The pathogenesis of the antiphospholipid syndrome. N Engl J Med 2013;368:1033–44.
7. Willis R, Harris EN, Pierangeli SS. Pathogenesis of the antiphospholipid syndrome. Semin Thromb Hemost 2012;38:305–21.
8. Lie JT. The distinction between vasculitis coincidental with and one that is causally related to the antiphospholipid syndrome. Arthritis Rheum 1992;35:1540.
9. Rocca PV, Siegel LB, Cupps TR. The concomitant expression of vasculitis and coagulopathy: synergy for marked tissue ischemia. J Rheumatol 1994;21:556–60.
10. Drenkard C, Villa AR, Reyes E, et al. Vasculitis in systemic lupus erythematous. Lupus 1997;6:235–42.
11. Love PE, Santoro SA. Antiphospholipid antibodies: anticardiolipin and the lupus anticoagulant in systemic lupus erythematosus (SLE) and in non-SLE disorders. Prevalence and clinical significance. Ann Intern Med 1990;112:682–98.
12. Ramos-Casals M, Nardi N, Lagrutta M, et al. Vasculitis in systemic lupus erythematosus: prevalence and clinical characteristics in 670 patients. Medicine (Baltimore) 2006;85:95–104.
13. Goldberger E, Elder RC, Schwartz RA, et al. Vasculitis in the antiphospholipid syndrome. A cause of ischemia responding to corticosteroids. Arthritis Rheum 1992;35:569–72.

14. Hansen KE, Moore KD, Ortel TL, et al. Antiphospholipid antibodies in patients with Wegener's granulomatosis and polyarteritis nodosa. Arthritis Rheum 1999;42:2250–2.

15. Cervera R, Piette JC, Font J, et al. Antiphospholipid syndrome: clinical and immunologic manifestations and patterns of disease expression in a cohort of 1,000 patients. Arthritis Rheum 2002;46:1019–27.

16. Thornsberry LA, LoSicco KI, English JC. The skin and hypercoagulable states. J Am Acad Dermatol 2013;69:450–62.

17. Francès C, Niang S, Laffitte E, et al. Dermatologic manifestations of the antiphospholipid syndrome: two hundred consecutive cases. Arthritis Rheum 2005;52:1785–93.

18. Acland KM, Darvay A, Wakelin SH, et al. Livedoid vasculitis: a manifestation of antiphospholipid syndrome? Br J Dermatol 1999;140:131–5.

19. Asherson RA, Jacobelli S, Rosenberg H, et al. Skin nodules and macules resembling vasculitis in the antiphospholipid syndrome—a report of two cases. Clin Exp Dermatol 1992;17:266–9.

20. Weinstein S, Piette W. Cutaneous manifestations of antiphospholipid antibody syndrome. Hematol Oncol Clin North Am 2008;22:67–77.

21. Kawakami T, Soma Y, Mizoguchi M. Initial cutaneous manifestations associated with histopathological leukocytoclastic vasculitis in two patients with antiphospholipid antibody syndrome. J Dermatol 2005;32:1032–7.

22. Tajima C, Suzuki Y, Mizushima Y, et al. Clinical significance of immunoglobulin A antiphospholipid antibodies: possible association with skin manifestations and small vessel vasculitis. J Rheumatol 1998;25:1730–6.

23. Utz VM, Tang J. Ocular manifestations of the antiphospholipid syndrome. Br J Ophthalmol 2011;95:454–9.

24. Asherson RA, Merry P, Acheson JF, et al. Antiphospholipid antibodies: a risk factor for occlusive ocular vascular disease in systemic lupus erythematosus and the 'primary' antiphospholipid syndrome. Ann Rheum Dis 1989;48:358–61.

25. Turaka K, Bryan JS, Kwong HM Jr, et al. Bilateral occlusive retinal vasculitis in a patient with primary antiphospholipid antibody syndrome. Can J Ophthalmol 2012;47:60–1.

26. Kurz DE, Wang RC, Kurz PA. Idiopathic retinal vasculitis, aneurysms, and neuroretinitis in a patient with antiphospholipid syndrome. Arch Ophthalmol 2012;130:257–8.

27. Miserocchi E, Baltatzis S, Foster CS. Ocular features associated with anticardiolipin antibodies: a descriptive study. Am J Ophthalmol 2001;131:451–6.

28. Gertner E. Diffuse alveolar hemorrhage in the antiphospholipid syndrome: spectrum of disease and treatment. J Rheumatol 1999;26:805–7.

29. Asherson RA, Cervera R, Wells AU. Diffuse alveolar hemorrhage: a nonthrombotic antiphospholipid lung syndrome? Semin Arthritis Rheum 2005;35:138–42.

30. Cartin-Ceba R, Peikert T, Ashrani A, et al. Primary antiphospholipid syndrome-associated diffuse alveolar hemorrhage. Arthritis Care Res (Hoboken) 2014; 66:301–10.

31. Deane KD, West SG. Antiphospholipid antibodies as a cause of pulmonary capillaritis and diffuse alveolar hemorrhage: a case series and literature review. Semin Arthritis Rheum 2005;35:154–65.

32. Espinosa G, Cervera R, Font J, et al. The lung in the antiphospholipid syndrome. Ann Rheum Dis 2002;61:195–8.

33. Toussirot E, Figarella-Branger D, Disdier P, et al. Association of cerebral vasculitis with a lupus anticoagulant. A case with brain pathology. Clin Rheumatol 1994;13:624–7.

34. Quintero M, Mirza N, Chang H, et al. Antiphospholipid antibody syndrome associated with primary angiitis of the central nervous system: report of two biopsy proven cases. Ann Rheum Dis 2006;65:408–9.
35. Jeruc J, Popovic M, Vizjak A, et al. Multiple mononeuropathy due to vasculitis associated with anticardiolipin antibodies: a case report. Folia Neuropathol 2006;44:140–3.
36. Rallings P, Exner T, Abraham R. Coronary artery vasculitis and myocardial infarction associated with antiphospholipid antibodies in a pregnant woman. Aust N Z J Med 1989;19:347–50.
37. Ames PR, Cianciaruso B, Bellizzi V, et al. Bilateral renal artery occlusion in a patient with primary antiphospholipid antibody syndrome: thrombosis, vasculitis or both? J Rheumatol 1992;19:1802–6.
38. Almeshari K, Alfurayh O, Akhtar M. Primary antiphospholipid syndrome and self-limited renal vasculitis during pregnancy: case report and review of the literature. Am J Kidney Dis 1994;24:505–8.
39. Jennette JC, Falk RJ, Bacon PA, et al. 2012 Revised International Chapel Hill Consensus Conference nomenclature of vasculitides. Arthritis Rheum 2013; 65:1–11.
40. Merkel PA, Chang Y, Pierangeli SS, et al. The prevalence and clinical associations of anticardiolipin antibodies in a large inception cohort of patients with connective tissue diseases. Am J Med 1996;101:576–83.
41. Handa R, Aggarwal P, Biswas A, et al. Microscopic polyangiitis associated with antiphospholipid syndrome. Rheumatology (Oxford) 1999;38:478–9.
42. Ferenczi K, Chang T, Camouse M, et al. A case of Churg-Strauss syndrome associated with antiphospholipid antibodies. J Am Acad Dermatol 2007;56: 701–4.
43. Castellino G, La Corte R, Santilli D, et al. Wegener's granulomatosis associated with antiphospholipid syndrome. Lupus 2000;9:717–20.
44. Shovman O, Langevitz P, Gilburd B, et al. Coincidence of granulomatosis and polyangiitis with atypical clinical manifestation and antiphospholipid syndrome. Lupus 2013;22:320–3.
45. Merkel PA, Lo GH, Holbrook JT, et al. Brief communication: high incidence of venous thromboembolic events among patients with Wegener's granulomatosis: the Wegener's clinical occurrence of thrombosis (WeCLOT) Study. Ann Intern Med 2005;142:620–6.
46. Weidner S, Hafezi-Rachti S, Rupprecht HD. Thromboembolic events as a complication of antineutrophil cytoplasmic antibody-associated vasculitis. Arthritis Rheum 2006;55:146–9.
47. Sebastian JK, Voetsch B, Stone JH, et al. The frequency of anticardiolipin antibodies and genetic mutations associated with hypercoagulability among patients with Wegener's granulomatosis with and without a history of a thrombotic event. J Rheumatol 2007;34:2446–50.
48. Lamprecht P, deGroot K, Schnabel A, et al. Anticardiolipin antibodies and antibodies to beta(2)-glycoprotein I in patients with Wegener's granulomatosis. Rheumatology (Oxford) 2000;39:568–70.
49. von Scheven E, Lu TT, Emery HM, et al. Thrombosis and pediatric Wegener's granulomatosis: acquired and genetic risk factors for hypercoagulability. Arthritis Rheum 2003;49:862–5.
50. Steen KS, Peters MJ, Zweegman S, et al. Relapsing splenic vein thrombosis associated with antiphospholipid antibodies in a patient with Wegener granulomatosis. J Clin Rheumatol 2007;13:92–3.

51. Meyer MF, Schnabel A, Schatz H, et al. Lack of association between antiphospholipid antibodies and thrombocytopenia in patients with Wegener's granulomatosis. Semin Arthritis Rheum 2001;31:4–11.
52. Paul SN, Sangle SR, Bennett AN, et al. Vasculitis, antiphospholipid antibodies, and renal artery stenosis. Ann Rheum Dis 2005;64:1800–2.
53. Wiesner O, Russell KA, Lee AS, et al. Antineutrophil cytoplasmic antibodies reacting with human neutrophil elastase as a diagnostic marker for cocaine-induced midline destructive lesions but not autoimmune vasculitis. Arthritis Rheum 2004;50:2954–65.
54. Gulati S, Donato AA. Lupus anticoagulant and ANCA associated thrombotic vasculopathy due to cocaine contaminated with levamisole: a case report and review of the literature. J Thromb Thrombolysis 2012;34:7–10.
55. Gaburri PD, Chebli JM, Attalla A, et al. Colonic ulcers in propylthiouracil-induced vasculitis with secondary antiphospholipid syndrome. Postgrad Med J 2005;81:338–40.
56. Vereckel E, Krivan G, Reti M, et al. Anti-TNF-alpha-induced antiphospholipid syndrome manifested as necrotizing vasculitis. Scand J Rheumatol 2010;39: 175–7.
57. Casanueva B, Rodriguez-Valverde V, Merino J, et al. Increased IgA-producing cells in the blood of patients with active Henoch-Schönlein purpura. Arthritis Rheum 1983;26:854–60.
58. Kawasaki Y. The pathogenesis and treatment of pediatric Henoch-Schönlein purpura nephritis. Clin Exp Nephrol 2011;15:648–57.
59. Yang YH, Huang MT, Lin SC, et al. Increased transforming growth factor-beta (TGF-beta)-secreting T cells and IgA anti-cardiolipin antibody levels during acute stage of childhood Henoch-Schönlein purpura. Clin Exp Immunol 2000; 122:285–90.
60. Kawakami T, Watabe H, Mizoguchi M, et al. Elevated serum IgA anticardiolipin antibody levels in adult Henoch-Schönlein purpura. Br J Dermatol 2006;155:983–7.
61. Kawakami T, Yamazaki M, Mizoguchi M, et al. High titer of serum antiphospholipid antibody levels in adult Henoch-Schönlein purpura and cutaneous leukocytoclastic angiitis. Arthritis Rheum 2008;59:561–7.
62. Kimura S, Takeuchi S, Soma Y, et al. Raised serum levels of interleukins 6 and 8 and antiphospholipid antibodies in an adult patient with Henoch-Schönlein purpura. Clin Exp Dermatol 2013;38:730–6.
63. Liu A, Zhang H. Detection of antiphospholipid antibody in children with Henoch-Schönlein purpura and central nervous system involvement. Pediatr Neurol 2012;47:167–70.
64. Asherson RA, Cervera R. Antiphospholipid antibodies and infections. Ann Rheum Dis 2003;62:388–93.
65. Basu N, Watts R, Bajema I, et al. EULAR points to consider in the development of classification and diagnostic criteria in systemic vasculitis. Ann Rheum Dis 2010;69:1744–50.
66. Allenbach Y, Seror R, Pagnoux C, et al. High frequency of venous thromboembolic events in Churg-Strauss syndrome, Wegener's granulomatosis and microscopic polyangiitis but not polyarteritis nodosa: a systematic retrospective study on 1130 patients. Ann Rheum Dis 2009;68:564–7.
67. Dasgupta B, Almond MK, Tanqueray A. Polyarteritis nodosa and the antiphospholipid syndrome. Br J Rheumatol 1997;36:1210–2.
68. Praderio L, D'Angelo A, Taccagni G, et al. Association of lupus anticoagulant with polyarteritis nodosa: report of a case. Haematologica 1990;75:387–90.

69. Egan AC, Caleyachetty R, Sabharwal T, et al. Endocarditis and ulnar artery aneurysm as presenting features of antiphospholipid syndrome and polyarteritis nodosa. Lupus 2005;14:914–7.

70. Valeyrie L, Bachot N, Roujeau JC, et al. Neurological manifestations of polyarteritis nodosa associated with the antiphospholipid syndrome. Ann Med Interne (Paris) 2003;154:479–82.

71. Schoonjans R, Van Vlem B, Weyers S, et al. Polyarteritis nodosa and the antiphospholipid syndrome. Clin Rheumatol 1996;15:410–3.

72. Musuruana JL, Cavallasca JA. Polyarteritis nodosa complicated by antiphospholipid syndrome. South Med J 2008;101:419–21.

73. Koutoulidis V, Chatziioannou A, Kostopoulos C, et al. Primary antiphospholipid syndrome: a unique presentation with multiple visceral aneurysms. Ann Rheum Dis 2005;64:1793–4.

74. Kawakami T, Yamazaki M, Misoguchi M, et al. High titer of anti-phosphatidylserine-prothrombin complex antibodies in patients with cutaneous polyarteritis nodosa. Arthritis Care Res 2007;57:1507–13.

75. Salvarani C, Crowson CS, O'Fallon WM, et al. Reappraisal of the epidemiology of giant cell arteritis in Olmstead County, Minnesota over a fifty-year period. Arthritis Rheum 2004;51:264–8.

76. Borg FA, Salter VL, Dasgupta B. Neuro-ophthalmic complications in giant cell arteritis. Curr Allergy Asthma Rep 2008;8:323–30.

77. Cid MC, Cervera R, Font J, et al. Recurrent arterial thrombosis in a patient with giant-cell arteritis and raised anticardiolipin antibody levels. Br J Rheumatol 1988;27:164–6.

78. Cid MC, Cervera R, Font J, et al. Late thrombotic events in patients with temporal arteritis and anticardiolipin antibodies. Clin Exp Rheumatol 1990;8:359–63.

79. McHugh NJ, James IE, Plant GT. Anticardiolipin and antineutrophil antibodies in giant cell arteritis. J Rheumatol 1991;17:916–22.

80. Espinoza LR, Jara LJ, Silveira LH, et al. Anticardiolipin antibodies in polymyalgia rheumatica-giant cell arteritis: association with severe vascular complications. Am J Med 1991;90:474–8.

81. Duhaut P, Berruyer M, Pinede L, et al. Anticardiolipin antibodies and giant cell arteritis: a prospective, multicenter case-control study. Groupe de Recherche sur l'Artérite à Cellules Géantes. Arthritis Rheum 1998;41:701–9.

82. Liozon E, Roussel V, Roblot P, et al. Absence of anti-beta2 glycoprotein I antibodies in giant cell arteritis: a study of 45 biopsy-proven cases. Br J Rheumatol 1998;37:1129–31.

83. Meyer O, Nicaise P, Moreau S, et al. Antibodies to cardiolipin and beta 2 glycoprotein I in patients with polymyalgia rheumatica and giant cell arteritis. Rev Rhum Engl Ed 1996;63:241–7.

84. Manna R, Latteri M, Cristiano G, et al. Anticardiolipin antibodies in giant cell arteritis and polymyalgia rheumatica: a study of 40 cases. Br J Rheumatol 1998;37:208–10.

85. Liozon E, Roblot P, Paire D, et al. Anticardiolipin antibody levels predict flares and relapses in patients with giant-cell (temporal) arteritis. A longitudinal study of 58 biopsy-proven cases. Rheumatology (Oxford) 2000;39:1089–94.

86. Le Tonquèze M, Dueymes M, Giovangrandi Y, et al. The relationship of anti-endothelial cell antibodies to anti-phospholipid antibodies in patients with giant cell arteritis and/or polymyalgia rheumatica. Autoimmunity 1995;20(1):59–66.

87. Cuchacovich R, Espinoza LR. Is antiphospholipid antibody determination clinically relevant to the vasculitides? Semin Arthritis Rheum 2001;31:1–3.

88. Kerr GS, Hallahan CW, Giordano J, et al. Takayasu arteritis. Ann Intern Med 1994;120:919–29.
89. Nava A, Senécal JL, Bañales JL, et al. Absence of antiphospholipid/co-factor antibodies in Takayasu arteritis. Int J Cardiol 2000;75:S99–104.
90. Park MC, Park YB, Jung SY, et al. Anti-endothelial cell antibodies and antiphospholipid antibodies in Takayasu's arteritis: correlations of their titers and isotype distributions with disease activity. Clin Exp Rheumatol 2006;24:S10–6.
91. Misra R, Aggarwal A, Chag M, et al. Raised anticardiolipin antibodies in Takayasu's arteritis. Lancet 1994;43:1644–5.
92. Nityanand S, Mishra K, Shrivastava S, et al. Autoantibodies against cardiolipin and endothelial cells in Takayasu's arteritis: prevalence and isotype distribution. Br J Rheumatol 1997;36:923–4.
93. Santiago MB, Paz O. Rare association of antiphospholipid syndrome and Takayasu arteritis. Clin Rheumatol 2007;26:821–2.
94. Fain O, Mathieu E, Seror O, et al. Aortitis: a new manifestation of primary antiphospholipid syndrome. Br J Rheumatol 1995;34:686–7.
95. Dhaon P, Das SK, Saran RK, et al. Is aorto-arteritis a manifestation of primary antiphospholipid antibody syndrome? Lupus 2011;20:1554–6.
96. Seror O, Fain O, Dordea M, et al. Aortitis with antiphospholipid antibodies: CT and MR findings. Eur Radiol 1998;8:1373–5.
97. Kaku B, Higuchi T, Kanaya H, et al. Usefulness of fluorine-18-fluorodeoxyglucose positron emission tomography in a patient with Takayasu's arteritis associated with antiphospholipid syndrome. Int Heart J 2006;47:311–7.
98. Hamuryudan V, Er T, Seyahi E, et al. Pulmonary artery aneurysms in Behçet syndrome. Am J Med 2004;117:867–70.
99. Tomasson G, Monach PA, Merkel PA. Thromboembolic disease in vasculitis. Curr Opin Rheumatol 2009;21:41–6.
100. Hatemi G, Yazici Y, Yazici H. Behçet's syndrome. Rheum Dis Clin North Am 2013;39:245–61.
101. Hull RG, Harris EN, Gharavi AE, et al. Anticardiolipin antibodies: occurrence in Behçet's syndrome. Ann Rheum Dis 1984;43:746–8.
102. Pereira RM, Gonçalves CR, Bueno C, et al. Anticardiolipin antibodies in Behçet's syndrome: a predictor of a more severe disease. Clin Rheumatol 1989;8:289–91.
103. Tokay S, Direskeneli H, Yurdakul S, et al. Anticardiolipin antibodies in Behçet's disease: a reassessment. Rheumatology (Oxford) 2001;40:192–5.
104. Shaker O, Ay El-Deen MA, El Hadidi H, et al. The role of heat shock protein 60, vascular endothelial growth factor and antiphospholipid antibodies in Behçet disease. Br J Dermatol 2007;156:32–7.
105. Caramaschi P, Poli G, Bonora A, et al. A study on thrombophilic factors in Italian Behçet's patients. Joint Bone Spine 2010;77:330–4.
106. El-Ageb EM, Al-Maini MH, Al-Shukaily AK, et al. Clinical features of Behçet's disease in patients in the Sultanate of Oman; the significance of antiphospholipid antibodies? Rheumatol Int 2002;21:176–81.

Advances in the Diagnosis of Large Vessel Vasculitis

Georgina Espígol-Frigolé, MD[a], Sergio Prieto-González, MD[a], Marco A. Alba, MD[a], Itziar Tavera-Bahillo, MD[a], Ana García-Martínez, MD[b], Rosa Gilabert, MD[c], José Hernández-Rodríguez, MD[a], Maria C. Cid, MD[a],*

KEYWORDS

- Giant-cell arteritis • Takayasu arteritis • Temporal artery biopsy • Imaging
- Diagnosis

KEY POINTS

- Temporal artery biopsy is the most sensitive and specific procedure for the diagnosis of giant-cell arteritis.
- Imaging techniques including color-duplex ultrasonography, computed tomography angiography, magnetic resonance angiography and positron emission tomography are emerging as useful diagnostic techniques by exploring additional vascular territories both in giant-cell arteritis and in Takayasu arteritis.
- Imaging may have a role in assessing disease activity and response to therapy that deserves to be further investigated.

INTRODUCTION

Primary large vessel vasculitides (LVVs) are granulomatous inflammatory conditions involving large and medium-sized arteries and include 2 related but distinct entities: giant-cell arteritis (GCA) and Takayasu arteritis (TAK).[1–3] Both conditions have remarkable anatomic and histopathologic similarities but also have substantial differences, mainly in demographic characteristics,[3–5] disease distribution,[6,7] and response to therapy.[2,3,8] GCA predominates in elderly white people, particularly in native peoples or descendants from northern Europe, whereas TAK primarily occurs in young women and is more frequent among people of Asian or Native American ancestry. In addition, the spectrum of artery sizes targeted by GCA seems to be broader than that affected

Supported by Ministerio de Economía y Competitividad (SAF 11/30073).

a Vasculitis Research Unit, Department of Systemic Autoimmune Diseases, Hospital Clínic, Institut d'Investigacions Biomèdiques August Pi I Sunyer (IDIBAPS), University of Barcelona, Villarroel 170, Barcelona 08036, Spain; b Vasculitis Research Unit, Emergency Department, Hospital Clínic, Institut d'Investigacions Biomèdiques August Pi I Sunyer (IDIBAPS), Villarroel 170, Barcelona 08036, Spain; c Center for Diagnostic Imaging, Hospital Clínic, Institut d'Investigacions Biomèdiques Pi i Sunyer (IDIBAPS), University of Barcelona, Villarroel 170, Barcelona 08036, Spain
* Corresponding author. Vasculitis Research Unit, Department of Systemic Autoimmune Diseases, Hospital Clínic, Villarroel 170, Barcelona 08036, Spain.
E-mail address: mccid@clinic.ub.es

Rheum Dis Clin N Am 41 (2015) 125–140
http://dx.doi.org/10.1016/j.rdc.2014.10.001
0889-857X/15/$ – see front matter © 2015 Elsevier Inc. All rights reserved.

rheumatic.theclinics.com

by TAK.[6] Although TAK usually affects the aorta and its primary and secondary tributaries, the spectrum of vascular involvement by GCA ranges from the aorta to small epicranial arteries and small arteries supplying the optic nerve and retina (**Fig. 1**).[6,7,9,10] Moreover, large vessel involvement is subclinical in most patients with GCA, in whom combinations of cranial, polymyalgic, or systemic symptoms dominate the clinical picture.[2] Development of symptomatic stenoses in large or medium-sized vessels is uncommon in GCA.[6,11] In contrast, typical TAK features are related to symptomatic stenosis of the primary or secondary branches of the aorta.[3,8]

The characteristic involvement of the epicranial arteries facilitates the histopathologic diagnosis of GCA, which is usually obtained through superficial temporal artery biopsy (TAB).[1,2] When performed in optimal conditions, TAB has a remarkable sensitivity and provides the most definitive diagnosis of GCA. However, a TAB is not always feasible and, occasionally, the superficial temporal artery may not be involved. Imaging in its various modalities, including color duplex ultrasonography (CDUS), contrast-enhanced computed tomography (CT) with or without CT angiography (CTA), magnetic resonance imaging (MRI) with or without angiography (MRA), and positron emission tomography (PET) with or without CT (PET/CT),[12] are emerging as seminal procedures for the diagnosis and evaluation of disease extent in patients with GCA. In TAK, diagnosis almost invariably relies on imaging techniques because of the inaccessibility of involved vessels.

Temporal Artery Biopsy

TAB is the gold standard for GCA diagnosis by showing the typical histopathologic findings, namely mononuclear cell infiltration of the artery wall (see **Fig. 1**).[13,14] Giant cells are present in more than 50% of biopsies but their presence is not mandatory to establish the histopathologic diagnosis of GCA. Additional features, including fragmentation of the internal elastic lamina and intimal hyperplasia, are typical but not sufficient to confirm the diagnosis in the absence of inflammatory infiltrates. To improve the diagnostic accuracy of the TAB, several issues need to be considered.

Reducing unnecessary biopsies
About 70% of TABs performed in referral centers are negative. In most patients an alternative diagnosis is obtained after additional work-up. As a result, in a substantial proportion of patients TAB could be avoided.[15–18] Several investigators have analyzed clinical data associated with TAB results. The absence of manifest or subtle cranial symptoms or abnormalities at the careful temporal artery examination is associated with low

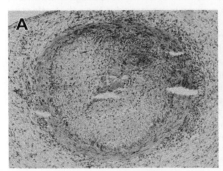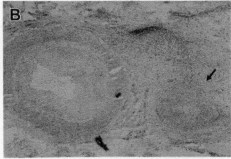

Fig. 1. Histopathologic findings in temporal artery biopsies from patients with GCA. (*A*) Typical transmural inflammation with disruption of the elastic lamina and lumen reduction by intimal hyperplasia. (*B*) Spared temporal artery with a clearly inflamed branch (*arrow*).

probability of a positive TAB even in patients who really have GCA.[15–18] In these cases other diagnostic approaches may achieve higher yield. However, a negative biopsy may be clinically helpful in driving attention toward other potential diagnoses. Moreover, a negative TAB may have an important clinical value by reasonably ruling out a treatable disorder in pluripathologic geriatric patients with constitutional symptoms.

Improving temporal artery biopsy sensitivity

In about 10% to 15 % of patients with a negative biopsy GCA is still suspected and patients are treated accordingly in spite of the TAB results.[15–18] TAB may be mistakenly negative when it is not performed or examined in optimal conditions and its sensitivity may be enhanced by improving those conditions. Because lesions may not be homogeneously distributed along the temporal artery, a lengthy fragment must be excised to achieve the maximal diagnostic performance.[15,16,19] It has been suggested that a 0.5-cm length after formalin fixation may be sufficient[20] but better sensitivity is obtained with fragments 2 cm or longer.[20,21] Note that specimens contract around 20% or more after excision.[21] Multiple sectioning and careful examination of multiple sections is crucial to increase the sensitivity of the TAB because lesions may be segmental.

Awareness by the examining pathologists of subtle abnormalities is also crucial. Early inflammatory changes including infiltrates surrounding vasa vasorum or inflammation of periadventitial vessels surrounding a spared temporal artery must be considered as relevant findings supporting GCA diagnosis in an appropriate clinical context (**Fig. 2**).[10,22–24] Sometimes, these incomplete findings are the only abnormality observed, but in other instances further sectioning reveals more characteristic features.[10,22–24] However, incomplete findings may be equivocal: involvement of periadventitial vessels can be seen in other vasculitides affecting medium or small vessels (polyarteritis nodosa or anti-neutrophil cytoplasmic antibody (ANCA) associated vasculitis).[10,25] Furthermore, slight inflammatory changes in small vessels or vasa vasorum can be seen in severe chronic infections such as endocarditis or in malignancies, possibly as a result of pattern recognition–mediated activation of endothelial cells or systemic release of inflammatory mediators.[26,27] There is a gray diagnostic zone in specimens with slight inflammatory changes and, when these are observed, additional diseases must be considered and additional diagnostic work-up must be performed.

Several investigators have raised the question of whether performing bilateral TABs would increase the diagnostic sensitivity of TAB. Discordant results between TABs

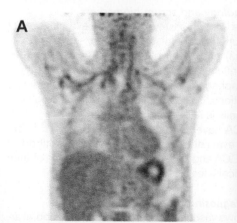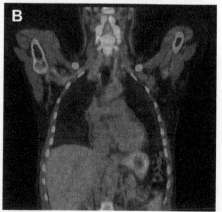

Fig. 2. Involvement of large vessels in GCA. (*A*) PET showing involvement of the supra-aortic branches and carotid arteries. (*B*) PET/CT from the same patient.

performed on both sides are obtained in 0% to 12.7% of cases according to various studies.[21,28–30] Therefore, routine performance of simultaneous bilateral TAB to increase diagnostic sensitivity is not advised, although performance of a second TAB when the first one is negative can be considered in particular patients with strong suspicion of GCA or in whom obtaining a definitive diagnostic confirmation is considered crucial.

When GCA is strongly suspected a prompt initiation of glucocorticoid treatment is advised, particularly in patients with visual symptoms. There has been some concern regarding how previous glucocorticoid treatment may influence the diagnostic accuracy of TAB by clearing inflammatory lesions. This relevant issue has been addressed in several studies. It seems clear that glucocorticoid treatment for a period of 8 weeks or less does not reduce the diagnostic yield of TAB.[31,32] However, over the months, lesions evolve to a healing or obsolescent stage with prominent fibrosis, vascular remodeling, and remaining scattered small foci of inflammatory cells.[14,33,34] In some patients this pattern is observed before the initiation of glucocorticoid treatment, perhaps suggesting that the disease may have started earlier than when clinically apparent.[14,34,35] Failure to recognize this pattern may also decrease the diagnostic performance of TAB.

Because TAB performance in optimal conditions and examination by expert and sensitized pathologists may not be invariably available, some investigators have emphasized the clinical diagnosis of GCA as the gold standard. Many investigators have used the 1990 American College of Rheumatology (ACR) classification criteria[36] or modified versions as diagnostic criteria, even in clinical trials.[37,38] However, the ACR criteria were not intended for this purpose and do not perform satisfactorily as diagnostic criteria.[39] Many conditions in elderly people convey headache, (i.e. anemia of any origin, depression) and moderate increase of acute-phase reactants and 3 ACR criteria can easily be fulfilled. In addition, about 10% to 20% of patients lack cranial symptoms and present with atypical features, such as fever of unknown origin, unexplained weight loss, or anemia of chronic disease type, and could never be diagnosed with GCA based exclusively on clinical grounds. Moreover, clinical diagnosis relies heavily on the experience of evaluating physicians and may have an important interobserver variability. Reported series of patients with GCA considered refractory to high-dose glucocorticoid treatment contain an exceedingly high rate of patients with negative/not performed biopsies, raising the question of whether some of these patients could have a mimicking disease.[40,41]

Diagnostic contribution of molecular pathology and serum biomarkers
Investigators have attempted to increase the sensitivity of routine examination of hematoxylin-eosin–stained slides by immunohistochemistry methods.

Immunostaining for T lymphocyte (CD3) and macrophage (CD68) markers may improve visualization and identification of inflammatory cells. However, small numbers of immunostained cells, particularly macrophages, may be observed in patients who are eventually diagnosed with other conditions.[28] The meaning of immunohistochemical detection of scattered inflammatory cells is still unclear.

Several inflammatory biomarkers of GCA have been identified in tissue[33,42,43] but their sensitivity and specificity needs to be evaluated. Circulating antiferritin antibodies have been detected in patients with both GCA and TAK.[44,45] The potential role of their detection in diagnosis needs to be specifically tested and validated.

The value of temporal artery biopsy in diagnosing other conditions
As mentioned earlier, TAB occasionally shows vascular inflammation in the temporal arteries or collateral branches in vasculitides other than GCA that may present with similar symptoms. Involvement of the temporal artery or its branches by ANCA-associated

vasculitis or polyarteritis nodosa has repeatedly been reported. TAB sometimes discloses histopathologic features typical of other diseases that may present with clinical signs or symptoms similar to GCA. Amyloidosis, thromboangiitis obliterans, and Kimura disease have been described in temporal artery specimens.[46,47]

Imaging

Timely performance and examination of TAB in optimal conditions is not universally feasible. Moreover, superficial temporal arteries may not invariably be involved and, as discussed earlier, interpretation of TAB results has some limitations. Along with the development, improvement in resolution, and widespread use of imaging techniques, these limitations have led to an active investigation of the role of imaging techniques in the diagnosis and assessment of patients with LVV.

Imaging may have various relevant roles in the evaluation of patients with LVV (**Box 1**). It may contribute to diagnosis of vascular inflammation by detecting thickening of the involved vessels or radiotracer uptake but it is also useful in assessing disease extent by exploring multiple vascular territories. Moreover, imaging may contribute to the evaluation of treatment efficacy and may constitute a valuable outcome measure, although this aspect has not been explored in depth. However, except for color duplex ultrasonography (CDUS), most existing studies consist of case reports, small series, or post hoc or retrospective analysis including heterogeneous patients in different activity states. Prospective, controlled studies using MRA, CTA, or PET are still scarce and distinct aspects such as diagnosis, extent, evaluation of disease activity, response to treatment, and damage/scarring have not been clearly defined or specifically addressed.

Imaging for large vessel vasculitis diagnosis

Imaging has always been the cornerstone of TAK diagnosis because histopathologic confirmation is not usually feasible because of the inaccessibility of the primarily involved vessels. In the past decade, the relevance of imaging in the diagnosis of GCA has increasingly been appreciated. CDUS of the temporal artery has a remarkable sensitivity and specificity for the diagnosis of GCA, especially when hypoechoic edematous wall swelling (the so-called halo sign) is detected.[12] Many articles and 3 meta-analyses leading to similar conclusions support the usefulness of CDUS for the diagnosis of GCA.[48–50] An advantage of CDUS compared with TAB is the potential assessment of longer artery segments or additional vascular beds. CDUS has shown that the axillary arteries are frequently involved in GCA and that distal extremity arteries such as ulnar or popliteal arteries may also be involved.[12,51–53] A recent study has shown that assessment of the axillary and common carotid arteries in addition to the temporal arteries may improve the diagnostic performance of CDUS.[54] It has been hypothesized that CDUS-guided selection of the temporal artery segment to be excised may increase the sensitivity of the TAB. However, a recent prospective, randomized study found that CDUS-guided TAB did not result in a higher rate of positive results than TAB guided by physical examination.[55]

A disadvantage of CDUS compared with TAB is the failure to detect slight histopathologic abnormalities such as periadventitial small vessel vasculitis or vasa vasorum vasculitis. In a recent study, the frequency of detection of the halo sign by CDUS was significantly lower in patients with incomplete histopathologic findings compared with those with classic transmural inflammation.[56]

High-resolution MRI has a sensitivity and specificity similar to CDUS in detecting temporal artery involvement in GCA,[57,58] although its routine use for this purpose is not widely feasible. A recent multicenter prospective study showed that

---

Box 1
Role of imaging in its various modalities in various steps of the assessment of patients with LVV (GCA and Takayasu arteritis)

Diagnosis

  Demonstration of temporal artery involvement in GCA

    CDUS

    MRI

  Evidence of LVV in both GCA and Takayasu arteritis

    CDUS: supra-aortic branches and extremity arteries

    PET: aorta and major tributaries

    MRA/CTA: aorta and major branches. Extremity arteries.

Evaluation of disease extent[a]

  CDUS: supra-aortic branches and extremity arteries

  PET: aorta and major tributaries

  MRA/CTA: aorta and major branches. Extremity arteries

  MRA/CTA/conventional angiography of coronary or intracranial arteries in selected patients

Detection of consequences of vascular remodeling

  Aortic/aortic branch dilatation or aneurysm (CT/MRI)

  Vascular stenoses (CTA, MRA, conventional angiography)

Evaluation of response to treatment (outcome measure)[b]

  CDUS

  PET

  CTA/MRA

  CEUS

Therapeutic intervention

  Conventional angiography (angioplasty ± stenting)

Abbreviations: CDUS, color duplex ultrasonography; CEUS, contrast-enhanced ultrasonography.
[a] Pattern of involvement may be useful in differentiating from other diseases (ie, periaortitis, isolated aortitis, vascular involvement by immunoglobulin G4 disease).
[b] Promising role but no definitive data are available.

---

high-resolution MRI has a sensitivity of 78.4% and a specificity of 90.4% in detecting temporal artery involvement in patients with clinical diagnosis of GCA, and a sensitivity of 88.7% and specificity of 75% using biopsy-proven disease as a reference.[58] In addition, MRI may detect deep temporal artery and temporalis muscle involvement in 20% to 40% of patients.[59] Considering these newly described abnormalities may increase the diagnostic yield of MRI.

PET takes advantage of increased metabolism in inflamed tissues and permits the noninvasive assessment of inflammation of the aorta and its tributaries (see **Fig. 2**).[52] When added to conventional evaluation of patients with suspected LVV, PET data influence clinical judgment and treatment decisions, and may increase diagnostic accuracy.[60]

In general, ^{18}F-fluorodeoxyglucose (FDG) uptake is considered to indicate vasculitis when the vascular signal is more intense than that of the liver.[12,52,61] However, increased FDG uptake can be seen in atheroma plaques and vascular aging and the threshold above which FDG uptake must be considered to indicate vascular inflammation is unclear.[61,62]

In order to calculate cutoffs with the best sensitivity and specificity by receiver-operator characteristic curve analysis, using an objective measure (maximal standardized uptake value [SUV_m]), a prospective case-control study including 32 newly diagnosed, biopsy-proven GCA and matched controls was performed.[63] Patients were imaged by PET/CT before or within the first 3 days after treatment onset.

The mean SUV_m was significantly higher in patients than in controls in all vessels explored (4 aortic segments, supra-aortic branches, and iliac-femoral territory). A cutoff of 1.89 for the mean of the SUV_m at all the vascular territories yielded a sensitivity and specificity of 80% and 79%, respectively, for LVV with an area under the curve of 0.830. If confirmed in larger studies, these findings may provide an objective and reproducible reference standard for LVV diagnosis by PET. A recent meta-analysis including 101 patients with GCA and 182 controls from 6 heterogeneous studies indicates a similar sensitivity (80%) and specificity (89%) for the diagnosis of LVV in GCA.[61]

CT and CTA are both useful for large vessel imaging because of their excellent spatial resolution and short scanning time. CT is useful in measuring aortic diameter in cases of dilatation and in detecting mural calcifications.[64–66] CTA may also assess concentric mural thickening, which is a characteristic finding of LVV.[11] Moreover, pre-contrast CT scanning shows mural thickening of high attenuation compared with the lumen, whereas in postcontrast-enhanced CTA images, a double ring in the venous phase is apparent.[11] The inside ring probably reflects intimal hyperplasia, whereas the outside ring indicates active inflammation in the adventitial and medial layers of the artery. Although ionizing radiation is of concern when successive explorations are necessary, new CT low-dose techniques and reconstruction systems provide substantial radiation reduction.[66]

MRI has higher resolution for soft tissues than CT or CTA but the spatial resolution is inferior. Like CTA, MRI can show mural thickening and may detect the presence of edema in T2 sequences. Moreover, MRA provides luminal information, including stenosis or dilatation, with no need for iodinated contrast or ionizing radiation and, for this reason, is the preferred technique for periodic assessment of patients with TAK.[67,68]

Assessing disease extent

Imaging in its various modalities has allowed the noninvasive appraisal of disease extension in LVV. For decades the involvement of the aorta and its branches in GCA was sporadically reported in necropsy or surgical reports of repaired aneurysms.[69,70] Involvement of large arteries detected by imaging (PET, CTA, or MRA) has subsequently been repeatedly reported in case reports or small case series.[71] Until recently the frequency of LVV in unselected patients with GCA was unknown. The first study assessing radiological signs of aortitis detected by CT was performed in a cohort of 22 patients with GCA imaged during the first month after diagnosis and assembled during a 10-year period.[72] Wall thickening was detected in the thoracic or abdominal aorta in 45% and 27% of patients, respectively. More recently, a larger prospective study analyzing 40 newly diagnosed patients with GCA by CTA before or within the first 3 days after the onset of glucocorticoid treatment disclosed vascular thickening in the aorta or its tributaries in up to 67.5% of patients with GCA (**Fig. 3**).[11] The most affected segments seem to be the aortic arch, the descending thoracic aorta, and the supra-aortic arteries.

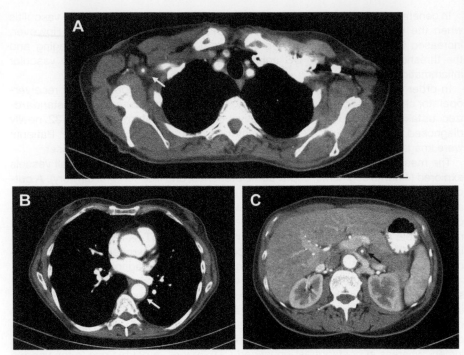

Fig. 3. CTA shows thickening of large vessel walls in GCA. (*A*) Right axillary artery (*arrow*), (*B*) descending aorta (*arrow*), (*C*) mesenteric artery (*arrow*).

Distribution of lesions in large vessels is similar among patients with GCA and TAK. However, detailed analysis of imaging has detected some differences.[7] In TAK, involvement of the left carotid artery and mesenteric artery is more frequent than in GCA, whereas in GCA involvement of the axillary arteries is significantly more common (see **Figs. 2** and **3**; **Fig. 4**). By cluster analysis it seems to be a transition group between the typical distribution of GCA lesions and that of TAK in patients with LVV younger than 55 years.

Medium artery involvement

Medium-sized arteries, defined as intraparenchymal visible arteries,[1] may be affected by LVV and can be an important source of morbidity and mortality.

Intracranial arteries can be involved in GCA and involvement of the carotid or vertebral branches may lead to ischemic stroke in 3% to 6% of patients (**Fig. 5**).[73,74] The frequency of such involvement is not well known because imaging is usually performed on symptomatic individuals only. MRA and conventional angiography allow the performance of angioplasty when necessary and have been the most frequently used techniques. In the carotid artery territory, the involvement of the carotid siphon has repeatedly been reported (see **Fig. 5**).[74,75] In a retrospective study performed with 50 patients with GCA, ophthalmic arteries were affected in 46% of patients. Involvement was more frequent in patients with ocular symptoms or complications.[76]

CTA has detected a remarkable frequency of silent coronary involvement in TAK. Using 128-section dual-source CTA, a recent study including 111 patients disclosed coronary lesions in more than half of the patients.[77] Nonostial stenosis (36.9%), ostial stenosis (28%), and coronary aneurysms (8.1%) were the main radiological features.

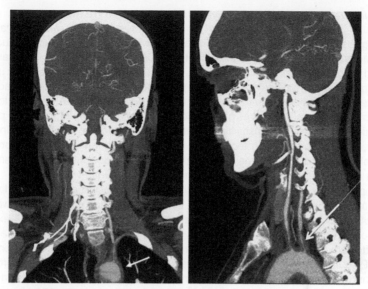

Fig. 4. Involvement of the aorta (*short arrow*) and the supra aortic branches (*long arrow*) with wall thickening and luminal narrowing in a patient with Takayasu arteritis. Front (*left*) and lateral (*right*) views of the same patient.

Effects of treatment on imaging findings

When imaging is used to assess patients with suspected LVV glucocorticoid treatment may quickly decrease the capacity of imaging to detect vascular inflammation. The halo sign frequently disappears 2 to 3 weeks after the initiation of glucocorticoid treatment,[78] but shorter treatment periods, even 2 to 3 days, may reduce its detection rate.[79,80] Brief treatment intervals may also reduce sensitivity with other imaging techniques such as CTA or MRI.[11,59,79,81] In contrast, in a recent study using PET/CT for assessment of large vessel inflammation in patients with newly diagnosed GCA[63] no significant differences in maximal or mean SUV_m were observed between treatment-naive patients and those who had received glucocorticoids for less than 3 days. However, longer periods of treatment seem to significantly decrease the diagnostic performance of PET.[60]

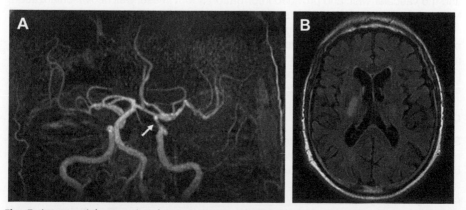

Fig. 5. Intracranial artery involvement in a patient with GCA. (*A*) MRA showing internal carotid artery stenosis (*arrow*) (*B*) T2-weighted MRI showing ischemic stroke.

Imaging in evaluation of disease activity and response to treatment
Changes in imaging findings induced by treatment suggest a role for imaging in assessing response to treatment and disease activity during follow-up. Evaluation of disease activity and response to treatment in GCA currently relies on clinical symptoms and laboratory abnormalities. In TAK, clinical symptoms are frequently indolent and laboratory abnormalities may be less apparent. Assessment of disease activity is one of the major challenges in the management of patients with TAK and periodic imaging has been recommended as part of the follow-up assessment, because physical examination has a limited sensitivity for detecting large vessel involvement in LVV.[82] However, none of the imaging techniques have been validated for this purpose and distinguishing by imaging between active inflammation susceptible to treatment intensification or consequences of vascular remodeling is an unsolved question.

This important issue needs to be prospectively explored because existing data mostly come from retrospective or post hoc studies. In TAK, correlation of PET findings with clinical symptoms or laboratory markers is not always consistent.[83–85] Serial PET examination in a cohort of 35 patients with GCA revealed a semiquantitative decrease in FDG uptake after 3 months of treatment, but no further reduction at 6 months was seen. Moreover, PET results were not predictive of relapses in this study.[52] In TAK, the reported sensitivities and specificities of PET for assessment of disease activity ranges from 69% to 93% and 33% to 100%, respectively,[67,83–85] with a pooled sensitivity of 70.1% and specificity of 77.2% in a recent meta-analysis of small case series or retrospective studies.[86]

Late contrast enhancement by MRA is commonly observed in patients with TAK and may reflect inflammatory activity. However, it may also indicate fibrosis, because it can also be observed in patients in stable remission (**Fig. 6**).[68,87] In contrast with gadolinium, the intravenous contrast gadofosveset does not enhance fibrous tissue and Papa and colleagues[88] evaluated its effectiveness to assess inflammatory activity in 23 patients with TAK. There was significant correlation between vessel wall contrast enhancement and disease activity. This promising approach needs wider evaluation and confirmation.

Future techniques
New imaging approaches are emerging and may be useful in the evaluation of LVV. Microbubble contrast-enhanced ultrasonography (CEUS) is increasingly used for vascular imaging.[89–92] A prospective study, including 7 patients with LVV, compared CDUS with CEUS for the assessment of carotid artery inflammation.[93] Microbubble contrast improved the image quality and the definition of the border between the lumen and the vascular wall, and provided information about vessel wall neovascularization. Moreover, a case report suggests that CEUS abnormalities improve with treatment.[91]

[11C]-PK11195, a selective ligand of membrane receptors of activated macrophages, has been investigated to detect vascular inflammation using PET. A preliminary study including 6 patients with LVV (4 GCA and 2 TAK) detected increased [11C]-PK11195 uptake in the arterial wall compared with 9 controls.[94] Further studies are needed to confirm and expand these results.

CONCLUDING REMARKS

Substantial advances in the diagnosis of patients with LVV have been achieved in recent years. Several studies have contributed to improving the diagnostic accuracy of histopathologic examination, and the potential role of tissue or serum biomarkers, although still in its infancy, has begun to be investigated. Imaging is rapidly and successfully expanding and is likely to become a reliable outcome measure in coming years, although prospective and validation studies are required (**Box 2**). International collaboration will be seminal in achieving these important goals.[95,96]

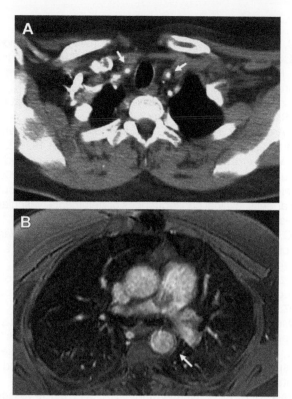

Fig. 6. Large vessel involvement in a patient with Takayasu disease in apparent clinical remission. (*A*) CTA showing artery wall thickening of the epiaortic branches (*arrows*). (*B*) Aortic wall thickening with delayed contrast enhancement (*arrow*).

Box 2
Conclusions/research agenda

1. Even with limitations, TAB provides the highest sensitivity and specificity for the diagnosis of GCA. Slight inflammatory changes are of diagnostic value. Other vasculitides occasionally involve the temporal artery or its branches, and TAB may reveal mimicking diseases.

2. Imaging techniques are emerging as highly valuable diagnostic tools and allow widespread evaluation of multiple vascular territories. Their diagnostic performance needs to be formally tested.

3. The performance of imaging in its present and emerging modalities in evaluating disease activity and response to treatments needs to be better evaluated in large and prospective studies

4. Improvement of imaging techniques is emerging by applying better contrast agents (ie, microbubbles for ultrasonography or gadofosveset for MRA) or by identifying more specific inflammation-related targets for PET scan.

5. Tissue-specific or serum-specific biomarkers with diagnostic significance need to be identified.

REFERENCES

1. Jennette JC, Falk RJ, Bacon PA, et al. 2012 revised International Chapel Hill Consensus Conference Nomenclature of Vasculitides. Arthritis Rheum 2013;65:1–11.
2. Salvarani C, Pipitone N, Versari A, et al. Clinical features of polymyalgia rheumatica and giant cell arteritis. Nat Rev Rheumatol 2012;8:509–21.
3. Maksimowicz-McKinnon K, Hoffman G. Takayasu arteritis: what is the long term prognosis? Rheum Dis Clin North Am 2007;33:777–86.
4. Michel BA, Arend WP, Hunder GG. Clinical differentiation between giant-cell (temporal) arteritis and Takayasu's arteritis. J Rheumatol 1996;23:106–11.
5. Magrey MN, Villa-Forte A, Koening CL, et al. Takayasu arteritis and giant-cell arteritis: a spectrum within the same disease? Medicine (Baltimore) 2009;88:221–6.
6. Cid MC, Prieto-González S, Arguis P, et al. The spectrum of vascular involvement in giant-cell arteritis: clinical consequences of detrimental vascular remodeling at different sites. APMIS 2009;117(Suppl):10–20.
7. Grayson PC, Maksimowicz-McKinnon K, Clark TM, et al, Vasculitis Clinical Research Consortium. Distribution of arterial lesions in Takayasu's arteritis and giant cell arteritis. Ann Rheum Dis 2012;71:1329–34.
8. Maksimowicz-McKinnon K, Clark TM, Hoffman GS. Limitations of therapy and a guarded prognosis in an American cohort of Takayasu arteritis patients. Arthritis Rheum 2007;56:1000–9.
9. Kattah JC, Mejico L, Chrousos GA, et al. Pathologic findings in a steroid –responsive optic nerve infarct in giant-cell arteritis. Neurology 1999;53:177–80.
10. Esteban MJ, Font C, Hernández-Rodríguez J, et al. Small vessel vasculitis surrounding a spared temporal artery: clinical and pathological findings in a series of 28 patients. Arthritis Rheum 2001;44:1387–95.
11. Prieto-González S, Arguis P, García-Martínez A, et al. Large vessel involvement in biopsy-proven giant cell arteritis: prospective study in 40 newly diagnosed patients using CT angiography. Ann Rheum Dis 2012;71:1170–6.
12. Blockmans D, Bley T, Schmidt W. Imaging for large-vessel vasculitis. Curr Opin Rheumatol 2009;21:19–28.
13. Lie JT. Illustrated histopathologic classification criteria for selected vasculitis syndromes. American College of Rheumatology Subcommittee on Classification of Vasculitis. Arthritis Rheum 1990;33:1074–87.
14. Lie JT. The classification and diagnosis of vasculitis in large and medium-sized blood vessels. Pathol Annu 1987;22(1):125–62.
15. Hall S, Persellin S, Lie JT, et al. The therapeutic impact of temporal artery biopsy. Lancet 1983;2(8361):1217–20.
16. Vilaseca J, González A, Cid MC, et al. Clinical usefulness of temporal artery biopsy. Ann Rheum Dis 1987;46:282–5.
17. Gonzalez-Gay MA, García-Porrua C, Llorca J, et al. Biopsy-negative giant cell arteritis: clinical spectrum and predictive factors for positive temporal artery biopsy. Semin Arthritis Rheum 2001;30:249–56.
18. Rodríguez-Pla A, Rosselló-Urgell J, Bosch-Gil JA, et al. Proposal to decrease the number of negative temporal artery biopsies. Scand J Rheumatol 2007;36:111–8.
19. Ypsilantis E, Courtney ED, Chopra N, et al. Importance of specimen length during temporal artery biopsy. Br J Surg 2011;98:1556–60.
20. Mahr A, Saba M, Kambouchner M, et al. Temporal artery biopsy for diagnosing giant cell arteritis: the longer, the better? Ann Rheum Dis 2006;65:826–8.
21. Breuer GS, Nesher R, Nesher G. Effect of biopsy length on the rate of positive temporal artery biopsies. Clin Exp Rheumatol 2009;27(1 Suppl 52):S10–3.

22. Belilos E, Maddox J, Kowalewski RM, et al. Temporal small-vessel inflammation in patients with giant cell arteritis: clinical course and preliminary immunohistopathologic characterization. J Rheumatol 2011;38:331–8.
23. Restuccia G, Cavazza A, Boiardi L, et al. Small-vessel vasculitis surrounding an uninflamed temporal artery and isolated vasa vasorum vasculitis of the temporal artery: two subsets of giant cell arteritis. Arthritis Rheum 2012;64:549–56.
24. Chatelain D, Duhaut P, Loire R, et al. Small-vessel vasculitis surrounding an uninflamed temporal artery: a new diagnostic criterion for polymyalgia rheumatica? Arthritis Rheum 2008;58:2565–73.
25. Généreau T, Lortholary O, Pottier MA, et al. Temporal artery biopsy: a diagnostic tool for systemic necrotizing vasculitis. French Vasculitis Study Group. Arthritis Rheum 1999;42:2674–81.
26. Lesser RS, Aledort D, Lie JT. Non-giant cell arteritis of the temporal artery presenting as the polymyalgia rheumatica-temporal arteritis syndrome. J Rheumatol 1995; 22:2177–82.
27. Curtiss LK, Tobias PS. Emerging role of Toll-like receptors in atherosclerosis. J Lipid Res 2009;50(Suppl):S340–5.
28. Zhou L, Luneau K, Weyand CM, et al. Clinicopathologic correlations in giant cell arteritis: a retrospective study of 107 cases. Ophthalmology 2009;116:1574–80.
29. Durling B, Toren A, Patel V, et al. Incidence of discordant temporal artery biopsy in the diagnosis of giant cell arteritis. Can J Ophthalmol 2014;49:157–61.
30. Boyev LR, Millar NR, Green WR. Efficacy of unilateral versus bilateral temporal artery biopsies for the diagnosis of giant cell arteritis. Am J Ophthalmol 1999;128:211–5.
31. Achkar AA, Lie JT, Hunder GG, et al. How does previous corticosteroid treatment affect the biopsy findings in giant cell (temporal) arteritis? Ann Intern Med 1994; 120:987–92.
32. Narváez J, Bernad B, Roig-Vilaseca D, et al. Influence of previous corticosteroid therapy on temporal artery biopsy yield in giant cell arteritis. Semin Arthritis Rheum 2007;37:13–9.
33. Visvanathan S, Rahman MU, Hoffman GS, et al. Tissue and serum markers of inflammation during the follow-up of patients with giant-cell arteritis–a prospective longitudinal study. Rheumatology (Oxford) 2011;50:2061–70.
34. Fauchald P, Rygvold O, Oystese B. Temporal arteritis and polymyalgia rheumatica. Clinical and biopsy findings. Ann Intern Med 1972;77:845–52.
35. Cavazza A, Muratore F, Boiardi L, et al. Inflamed temporal artery: histologic findings in 354 biopsies, with clinical correlations. Am J Surg Pathol 2014;38:1360–70.
36. Hunder GG, Bloch DA, Michel BA, et al. The American College of Rheumatology 1990 criteria for the classification of giant cell arteritis. Arthritis Rheum 1990;33: 1122–8.
37. Hoffman GS, Cid MC, Hellmann DB, et al. A multicenter, randomized, double-blind, placebo-controlled trial of adjuvant methotrexate treatment for giant cell arteritis. Arthritis Rheum 2002;46:1309–18.
38. Hoffman GS, Cid MC, Rendt-Zagar KE, et al, Infliximab-GCA Study Group. Infliximab for maintenance of glucocorticosteroid-induced remission of giant cell arteritis: a randomized trial. Ann Intern Med 2007;146:621–30.
39. Rao JK, Allen NB, Pincus T. Limitations of the 1990 American College of Rheumatology classification criteria in the diagnosis of vasculitis. Ann Intern Med 1998; 129:345–52.
40. Unizony S, Arias-Urdaneta L, Miloslavsky E, et al. Tocilizumab for the treatment of large-vessel vasculitis (giant cell arteritis, Takayasu arteritis) and polymyalgia rheumatica. Arthritis Care Res (Hoboken) 2012;64:1720–9.

41. Quartuccio L, Maset M, De Maglio G, et al. Role of oral cyclophosphamide in the treatment of giant cell arteritis. Rheumatology (Oxford) 2012;51:1677–86.
42. Weyand CM, Hicok KC, Hunder GG, et al. Tissue cytokine patterns in patients with polymyalgia rheumatica and giant cell arteritis. Ann Intern Med 1994; 121(7):484–91.
43. Lally L, Pernis A, Narula N, et al. Increased rho kinase activity in temporal artery biopsies from patients with giant cell arteritis. Rheumatology (Oxford) 2014. [Epub ahead of print].
44. Große K, Witte T, Moosig F, et al. Association of ferritin antibodies with Takayasu arteritis. Clin Rheumatol 2014;33:1523–6.
45. Monach PA. Biomarkers in vasculitis. Curr Opin Rheumatol 2014;26(1):24–30.
46. Azari AA, Kanavi MR, Girgis D, et al. Amyloid deposits in temporal artery mimicking temporal arteritis in a patient with multiple myeloma. JAMA Ophthalmol 2013;131:1488.
47. Cid MC, Campo E. Diagnostic efficacy of temporal artery biopsy. Med Clin (Barc) 1989;92(3):95–7.
48. Karassa FB, Matsagas MI, Schmidt WA, et al. Meta-analysis: test performance of ultrasonography for giant-cell arteritis. Ann Intern Med 2005;142:359–69.
49. Arida A, Kyprianou M, Kanakis M, et al. The diagnostic value of ultrasonography-derived edema of the temporal artery wall in giant cell arteritis: a second meta-analysis. BMC Musculoskelet Disord 2010;11:44.
50. Ball EL, Walsh SR, Tang TY, et al. Role of ultrasonography in the diagnosis of temporal arteritis. Br J Surg 2010;97:1765–71.
51. Schmidt WA, Seifert A, Gromnica-Ihle E, et al. Ultrasound of proximal upper extremity arteries to increase the diagnostic yield in large-vessel giant cell arteritis. Rheumatology (Oxford) 2008;47(1):96–101.
52. Blockmans D, de Ceuninck L, Vanderschueren S, et al. Repetitive 18F-fluorodeoxyglucose positron emission tomography in giant cell arteritis: a prospective study of 35 patients. Arthritis Rheum 2006;55:131–7.
53. Aschwanden M, Kesten F, Stern M, et al. Vascular involvement in patients with giant cell arteritis determined by duplex sonography of 2x11 arterial regions. Ann Rheum Dis 2010;69:1356–9.
54. Diamantopoulos AP, Haugeberg G, Hetland H, et al. Diagnostic value of color Doppler ultrasonography of temporal arteries and large vessels in giant cell arteritis: a consecutive case series. Arthritis Care Res (Hoboken) 2014;66: 113–9.
55. Germano G, Muratore F, Cimino L, et al. Is colour duplex sonography-guided temporal artery biopsy useful in the diagnosis of giant cell arteritis? A randomized study. Rheumatology (Oxford) 2014. [Epub ahead of print].
56. Muratore F, Boiardi L, Restuccia G, et al. Comparison between colour duplex sonography findings and different histological patterns of temporal artery. Rheumatology (Oxford) 2013;52:2268–74.
57. Bley TA, Reinhard M, Hauenstein C, et al. Comparison of duplex sonography and high-resolution magnetic resonance imaging in the diagnosis of giant cell (temporal) arteritis. Arthritis Rheum 2008;58:2574–8.
58. Klink T, Geiger J, Both M, et al. Giant cell arteritis: diagnostic accuracy of MR imaging of superficial cranial arteries in initial diagnosis-results from a multicenter trial. Radiology 2014;140056.
59. Veldhoen S, Klink T, Geiger J, et al. MRI displays involvement of the temporalis muscle and the deep temporal artery in patients with giant cell arteritis. Eur Radiol 2014;24(11):2971–9.

60. Fuchs M, Briel M, Daikeler T, et al. The impact of 18F-FDG PET on the management of patients with suspected large vessel vasculitis. Eur J Nucl Med Mol Imaging 2012;39:344–53.
61. Besson FL, Parienti JJ, Bienvenu B, et al. Diagnostic performance of (1)F-fluoro-deoxyglucose positron emission tomography in giant cell arteritis: a systematic review and meta-analysis. Eur J Nucl Med Mol Imaging 2011;38:1764–72.
62. Orellana MR, Bentourkia M, Sarrhini O, et al. Assessment of inflammation in large arteries with 18F-FDG-PET in elderly. Comput Med Imaging Graph 2013;37:459–65.
63. Prieto-González S, Depetris M, García-Martínez A, et al. Positron emission tomography assessment of large vessel inflammation in patients with newly diagnosed, biopsy-proven giant cell arteritis: a prospective, case-control study. Ann Rheum Dis 2014;73:1388–92.
64. García-Martínez A, Hernández-Rodríguez J, Arguis P, et al. Development of aortic aneurysm/dilatation during the followup of patients with giant cell arteritis: a cross-sectional screening of fifty-four prospectively followed patients. Arthritis Rheum 2008;59:422–30.
65. García-Martínez A, Arguis P, Prieto-González S, et al. Prospective long term follow-up of a cohort of patients with giant cell arteritis screened for aortic structural damage (aneurysm or dilatation). Ann Rheum Dis 2014;73:1826–32.
66. Alkadhi H, Schindera ST. State of the art low-dose CT angiography of the body. Eur J Radiol 2011;80:36–40.
67. Hartlage GR, Palios J, Barron BJ, et al. Multimodality imaging of aortitis. JACC Cardiovasc Imaging 2014;7:605–19.
68. Tso E, Flamm SD, White RD, et al. Takayasu arteritis: utility and limitations of magnetic resonance imaging in diagnosis and treatment. Arthritis Rheum 2002;46:1634–42.
69. Ostberg G. Temporal arteritis in a large necropsy series. Ann Rheum Dis 1971;30:224–35.
70. Lie JT. Aortic and extracranial large vessel giant cell arteritis: a review of 72 cases with histopathologic documentation. Semin Arthritis Rheum 1995;24:422–31.
71. Narváez J, Narváez JA, Nolla JM, et al. Giant cell arteritis and polymyalgia rheumatica: usefulness of vascular magnetic resonance imaging studies in the diagnosis of aortitis. Rheumatology (Oxford) 2005;44:479–83.
72. Agard C, Barrier JH, Dupas B, et al. Aortic involvement in recent-onset giant cell (temporal) arteritis: a case-control prospective study using helical aortic computed tomodensitometric scan. Arthritis Rheum 2008;59(5):670–6.
73. Gonzalez-Gay MA, Vazquez-Rodriguez TR, Gomez-Acebo I, et al. Strokes at time of disease diagnosis in a series of 287 patients with biopsy-proven giant cell arteritis. Medicine (Baltimore) 2009;88:227–35.
74. Solans-Laqué R, Bosch-Gil JA, Molina-Catenario CA, et al. Stroke and multi-infarct dementia as presenting symptoms of giant cell arteritis: report of 7 cases and review of the literature. Medicine (Baltimore) 2008;87:335–44.
75. Alba MA, Espígol-Frigolé G, Prieto-González S, et al. Central nervous system vasculitis: still more questions than answers. Curr Neuropharmacol 2011;9:437–48.
76. Geiger J, Ness T, Uhl M, et al. Involvement of the ophthalmic artery in giant cell arteritis visualized by 3T MRI. Rheumatology (Oxford) 2009;48:537–41.
77. Kang EJ, Kim SM, Choe YH, et al. Takayasu arteritis: assessment of coronary arterial abnormalities with 128-section dual-source CT angiography of the coronary arteries and aorta. Radiology 2014;270:74–81.
78. Schmidt WA. Ultrasound in vasculitis. Clin Exp Rheumatol 2014;32:S71–7.

79. Hauenstein C, Reinhard M, Geiger J, et al. Effects of early corticosteroid treatment on magnetic resonance imaging and ultrasonography findings in giant cell arteritis. Rheumatology (Oxford) 2012;51:1999–2003.
80. Santoro L, D'Onofrio F, Bernardi S, et al. Temporal ultrasonography findings in temporal arteritis: early disappearance of halo sign after only 2 days of steroid treatment. Rheumatology (Oxford) 2013;52:622.
81. Prieto-Gonzalez S, Garcia-Martinez A, Arguis P, et al. Early improvement of radiological signs of large-vessel inflammation in giant cell arteritis upon glucocorticoid treatment. Rheumatology (Oxford) 2013;52:1335–6.
82. Grayson PC, Tomasson G, Cuthbertson D, et al, Vasculitis Clinical Research Consortium. Association of vascular physical examination findings and arteriographic lesions in large vessel vasculitis. J Rheumatol 2012;39:303–9.
83. Treglia G, Mattoli MV, Leccisotti L, et al. Usefulness of whole-body fluorine-18-fluorodeoxyglucose positron emission tomography in patients with large-vessel vasculitis: a systematic review. Clin Rheumatol 2011;30:1265–75.
84. Tezuka D, Haraguchi G, Ishihara T, et al. Role of FDG PET-CT in Takayasu arteritis: sensitive detection of recurrences. JACC Cardiovasc Imaging 2012;5:422–9.
85. Lee KH, Cho A, Choi YJ, et al. The role of (18) F-fluorodeoxyglucose-positron emission tomography in the assessment of disease activity in patients with Takayasu arteritis. Arthritis Rheum 2012;64:866–75.
86. Cheng Y, Lv N, Wang Z, et al. 18-FDG-PET in assessing disease activity in Takayasu arteritis: a meta-analysis. Clin Exp Rheumatol 2013;31:S22–7.
87. Eshet Y, Pauzner R, Goitein O, et al. The limited role of MRI in long-term follow-up of patients with Takayasu's arteritis. Autoimmun Rev 2011;11:132–6.
88. Papa M, De Cobelli F, Baldissera E, et al. Takayasu arteritis: intravascular contrast medium for MR angiography in the evaluation of disease activity. AJR Am J Roentgenol 2012;198:W279–84.
89. Feinstein SB, Coll B, Staub D, et al. Contrast enhanced ultrasound imaging. J Nucl Cardiol 2010;17:106–15.
90. Ten Kate GL, van den Oord SC, Sijbrands EJ, et al. Current status and future developments of contrast-enhanced ultrasound of carotid atherosclerosis. J Vasc Surg 2013;57:539–46.
91. Giordana P, Baque-Juston MC, Jeandel PY, et al. Contrast-enhanced ultrasound of carotid artery wall in Takayasu disease: first evidence of application in diagnosis and monitoring of response to treatment. Circulation 2011;124:245–7.
92. Magnoni M, Dagna L, Coli S, et al. Assessment of Takayasu arteritis activity by carotid contrast-enhanced ultrasound. Circ Cardiovasc Imaging 2011;4:e1–2.
93. Schinkel AF, van den Oord SC, van der Steen AF, et al. Utility of contrast-enhanced ultrasound for the assessment of the carotid artery wall in patients with Takayasu or giant cell arteritis. Eur Heart J Cardiovasc Imaging 2014;15:541–6.
94. Pugliese F, Gaemperli O, Kinderlerer AR, et al. Imaging of vascular inflammation with [11C]-PK11195 and positron emission tomography/computed tomography angiography. J Am Coll Cardiol 2010;56:653–61.
95. Basu N, Watts R, Bajema I, et al. EULAR points to consider in the development of classification and diagnostic criteria in systemic vasculitis. Ann Rheum Dis 2010;69:1744–50.
96. Craven A, Robson J, Ponte C, et al. ACR/EULAR-endorsed study to develop diagnostic and classification criteria for vasculitis (DCVAS). Clin Exp Nephrol 2013;17:619–21.

Challenging Mimickers of Primary Systemic Vasculitis

Eli M. Miloslavsky, MD, John H. Stone, MD, MPH*, Sebastian H. Unizony, MD

KEYWORDS

- Mimicker • Vasculitis • IgG4-related disease • Livedoid vasculopathy
- Segmental arterial mediolysis • Lymphomatoid granulomatosis
- Fibromuscular dysplasia • Degos disease

KEY POINTS

- Immunoglobulin G4–related disease is a common mimicker of small vessel and medium vessel vasculitides, particularly granulomatosis with polyangiitis, but it can also cause a true vasculitis of large vessels, requiring distinction from giant cell arteritis, among other vasculitides.
- Arterial instrumentation should be avoided whenever possible in cases of segmental arterial mediolysis and fibromuscular dysplasia, because such procedures can lead to arterial dissections.
- Calciphylaxis typically involves adipose tissues (eg, the thighs, buttocks, abdomen, and flanks).
- The myeloproliferative form of hypereosinophilic syndrome can be detected with examination of the bone marrow in addition to blood or bone marrow aspirate testing for FIP1L1/PDGFRA fusion, which is present in a subset of such patients.
- Of livedoid vasculitis begin as tender erythematous nodules that then rapidly ulcerate and scar with atrophie blanche. The ulcers have an irregular shape and are extremely painful.

Among the most challenging aspects of evaluating and caring for patients with systemic vasculitis is the need to distinguish rigorously between vasculitis and a host of conditions that can mimic vasculitis closely (**Box 1**). The treatment approaches for vasculitis mimickers are varied and often differ substantially from those required to treat vasculitis. This article reviews 9 challenging vasculitis mimickers: fibromuscular dysplasia (FMD), calciphylaxis, segmental arterial mediolysis, antiphospholipid syndrome (APS), hypereosinophilic syndrome, lymphomatoid granulomatosis (LMPG), malignant atrophic papulosis, livedoid vasculopathy, and immunoglobulin (Ig) G4–related disease (IgG4-RD).

Rheumatology Unit, Massachusetts General Hospital, Yawkey 2, 55 Fruit Street, Boston, MA 02114, USA
* Corresponding author.
E-mail address: jhstone@mgh.harvard.edu

Rheum Dis Clin N Am 41 (2015) 141–160
http://dx.doi.org/10.1016/j.rdc.2014.09.011
0889-857X/15/$ – see front matter © 2015 Elsevier Inc. All rights reserved.

rheumatic.theclinics.com

> **Box 1**
> **Systemic vasculitis mimickers: a comprehensive list**
>
> Conditions mimicking small vessel vasculitis
>
>   Antiphospholipid antibody syndrome[a]
>
>   Atheroembolic disease
>
>   Calciphylaxis[a]
>
>   Hypereosinophilic syndrome[a]
>
>   Emboli (cardiac myxoma, cardiac thrombus, endocarditis, mycotic aneurysm, others)
>
>   Idiopathic diffuse alveolar hemorrhage
>
>   Infection (endocarditis, disseminated intravascular coagulation, Rocky Mountain spotted fever, others)
>
>   Intravascular lymphoma
>
>   Levamisole-induced vasculitis
>
>   Lymphomatoid granulomatosis[a]
>
>   Malignant atrophic papulosis (Degos disease)[a]
>
>   Thrombotic thrombocytopenic purpura[a]
>
> Conditions mimicking medium vessel vasculitis
>
>   Livedoid vasculopathy[a]
>
>   Fibromuscular dysplasia[a]
>
>   Segmental arterial mediolysis[a]
>
>   Thromboangiitis obliterans (Buerger disease)
>
> Conditions mimicking large vessel vasculitis
>
>   IgG4-related disease[a]
>
>   Erdheim-Chester disease
>
>   Ehlers-Danlos type IV
>
>   Loeys-Dietz syndrome
>
>   Marfan syndrome
>
> Conditions affecting a single organ
>
>   Reversible cerebral vasoconstriction syndrome[a]
>
>   [a] Discussed in this article.

FIBROMUSCULAR DYSPLASIA

FMD is a noninflammatory vasculopathy of small and medium-sized arteries that can lead to aneurysm, stenosis, occlusion, and dissection.[1,2] This disease may occur in any age group, but mainly affects children and individuals more than 50 years of age.[3,4] The prevalence of FMD in the general population is estimated to be around 2% to 3%.[4,5] Women comprise up to 90% of cases in adults.[3,6] Approximately 10% of patients with FMD report a family member carrying the same diagnosis.[3,7]

The most commonly affected vascular sites are middle and distal portions of the renal, internal carotid, and vertebral arteries (~65% of the cases).[3] Lesions are detected less frequently in the intracranial, common carotid, external carotid, subclavian, coronary, mesenteric, iliac, and limb arteries.[3,8] Aortic disease has rarely been reported. More than half of the patients have 2 or more vascular territories involved, and bilateral distributions of disease are common.[4] The etiopathogenesis of FMD is poorly understood, but genetic, biomechanical, and hormonal factors have been implicated.[9]

FMD is classified in 5 main types, based on the histologic characteristics and the location of the process within the arterial wall. These types are: (1) medial fibroplasia (~90%), (2) intimal fibroplasia (~10%), (3) perimedial fibroplasia (<1%), (4) medial hyperplasia (<1%), and (5) adventitial (periarterial) hyperplasia (<1%).[5] The specific FMD type correlates well with the radiologic findings in a given case (discussed later).

The presentation of FMD is determined primarily by the distribution of the arteries that are involved. The presentations vary from incidental findings in asymptomatic individuals to a diverse array of clinical manifestations such as renovascular hypertension (the most common presentation), headache, lightheadedness, pulsatile tinnitus, neck pain, limb claudication, postprandial angina, and acute coronary syndrome.[3,5,6,10] The physical examination may reveal pulse deficits, asymmetric blood pressure readings, and vascular bruits. At times, patients present with rupture of an aneurysm (eg, subarachnoid hemorrhage). Embolization of intravascular thrombi from aneurysmal segments can also occur, leading to amaurosis fugax, transient ischemic attack, stroke, and cyanotic toes.[3] Spontaneous arterial dissections, most frequently of the carotid arteries, occur in up to 20% of the patients.[3] Arterial aneurysms are seen in approximately 20% of the cases as well. Both dissections and aneurysms seem to be more prevalent in men.[11]

The diagnosis of FMD is typically made with vascular imaging. Duplex ultrasonography is a reasonable first-line screening technique, followed by noninvasive studies such as computed tomography angiography (CTA) or magnetic resonance angiography (MRA) as confirmatory tests. However, conventional angiography remains the gold standard for diagnosis.[5] The classic string-of-beads appearance on angiography generally corresponds with the medial fibroplasia FMD type (**Fig. 1**). In contrast, unifocal lesions described as focal concentric narrowing and diffuse tubular stenosis correlate more closely with the intimal and periadventitial fibroplasia FMD types.[6]

The differential diagnoses of FMD from a rheumatologic perspective are Takayasu arteritis (TAK), giant cell arteritis (GCA), and polyarteritis nodosa (PAN). Clues that may help to differentiate FMD from vasculitides include the presence of normal inflammatory markers (unless severe ischemia leads to tissue infarction); the absence of arthralgias, fever or constitutional symptoms; and the absence of arterial wall thickening, edema, or contrast uptake on cross-sectional vascular imaging. On diagnosis, patients with FMD should undergo screening of the cervical, intracranial, and renal vasculature to identify potential synchronous lesions.[3,12]

The treatment of FMD may include medical therapy and surveillance, endovascular procedures, and surgery.[5] However, disease-modifying agents have not been identified. Patients with renovascular hypertension require antihypertensive therapy. Hypertension in this setting is secondary to upregulation of the renin-angiotensin-aldosterone system,[13] therefore the drugs of choice are angiotensin receptor blockers (ARBs) and angiotensin-converting enzyme inhibitors (ACEIs). Close monitoring of kidney function is required during the initiation of ARBs or ACEIs because a subset of patients with FMD develop abrupt decline in the glomerular filtration rate, requiring drug discontinuation. More than 1 pharmacologic agent is frequently needed for adequate blood pressure control.

For patients with hypertension who respond poorly to medical therapy or for those with hemodynamically significant lesions in the renal arteries or in other vascular

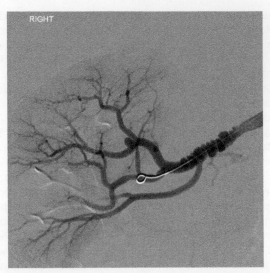

Fig. 1. Fibromuscular dysplasia. Conventional angiography in a patient with FMD showing a classic string-of-beads lesion affecting the distal portion of a right renal artery. (*Courtesy of* Dr George Oliveira, Massachusetts General Hospital.)

territories, revascularization is indicated. Endovascular treatment options include percutaneous transluminal balloon angioplasty (PTA) with or without stenting (eg, stenoses, dissections, and aneurysms) or coiling (eg, aneurysms). Surgical interventions are reserved for restenosis after PTA, complex lesions, or lesions that are difficult to reach by PTA (eg, renal artery branches). Unlike atherosclerotic disease, resolution of hypertension is common after revascularization of FMD-related renal artery stenosis.[14]

Monitoring via imaging is required after PTA or surgery to assess the short-term and long-term patency of revascularized arterial segments. If no revascularization is indicated, longitudinal imaging surveillance is also advisable to monitor the progression of disease and determine the indication and timing of revascularization. Experts recommend heparin therapy acutely followed by 3 to 6 months of anticoagulation with warfarin for patients who develop arterial dissection.[15] However, high-quality evidence supporting this practice is still not available.[16] In addition, identification and correction of concomitant cardiovascular risk factors (eg, smoking, dyslipidemia, and diabetes) is strongly recommended.[5]

CALCIPHYLAXIS

Calciphylaxis is a noninflammatory vasculopathy characterized by ectopic calcification within the wall of small and medium-sized arteries. This potentially serious process can lead to vascular occlusion, ischemia, and necrosis of the skin and subcutaneous tissues.[17] Calciphylaxis is observed in up to 4% of patients undergoing hemodialysis and is therefore sometimes termed calcific uremic arteriolopathy.[18] However, the disease can also occur in nonuremic patients.

Calciphylaxis has been described in the context of primary hyperparathyroidism, malignancy, chronic liver disease, acute kidney injury, inflammatory bowel disease, warfarin anticoagulation, and systemic autoimmune disorders (eg, systemic lupus erythematosus, Sjögren syndrome, polymyositis, rheumatoid arthritis, APS, sarcoidosis, and GCA).[19–22] The disease is usually seen in the fifth or sixth decade of life, and is most frequent in women.[22,23] Some studies indicate that obesity, hypoalbuminemia, and the use of corticosteroids are also risk factors.[17,19]

The etiopathogenesis of calciphylaxis is poorly understood. Disturbances of calcium-phosphate homeostasis are clearly central to the disease process, as shown by the increased prevalence in patients with end-stage renal disease (ESRD)[24] and parathyroid dysfunction. Moreover, parathyroid hormone (PTH) or vitamin D administration is known to induce soft tissue calcification and skin necrosis in experimental models.[25] Additional research suggests that deficiency of circulatory and tissue calcium and phosphate binding proteins (eg, fetuin-A, matrix Gla protein),[26,27] inflammation, and alteration of the coagulation (eg, protein C and S deficiency)[28] and the RANK (receptor activator of nuclear factor kappa-B)/osteoprotegerin systems[29] might also be involved in the pathogenesis of the disease.

Calciphylaxis typically involves adipose tissues (eg, the thighs, buttocks, abdomen, flanks). A variety of cutaneous lesions can be evident: violaceous, indurated plaques and nodules; ulcerations; necrotic eschars; and lesions that mimic the purpura of vasculitis (**Fig. 2**).[22] Skin lesions are extremely painful and easily become infected. Skin contractures, penile involvement, myopathy, or cardiopulmonary calcification may rarely develop.[30–32] The diagnosis is usually made by skin biopsy, which shows medial calcification, intimal hyperplasia, intimal fibrosis, and superimposed thrombosis affecting dermohypodermic arterioles and venules (**Fig. 3**). Vascular obstruction leads to ischemia, necrosis, and secondary inflammation (calcifying septal panniculitis).

In patients with ESRD, the serum levels of PTH, calcium, and/or phosphate tend to be increased. However, most nonuremic calciphylaxis cases have no obvious abnormalities of those parameters.[19] Radiography and computed tomography of the affected areas may reveal vascular and extravascular calcium deposits. In addition, 3-phase technetium methylene diphosphate bone scans can help to define the extension of the disease and also monitor response to therapy.[31,33] The differential diagnosis of calciphylaxis not only includes systemic necrotizing vasculitides (eg, PAN, cryoglobulinemia, and antineutrophil cytoplasmic antibody (ANCA) associated vasculitis),[22] but also warfarin-induced skin necrosis, primary skin and soft tissue infections, cholesterol atheroembolism, APS, neutrophilic dermatosis, and nephrogenic systemic fibrosis.

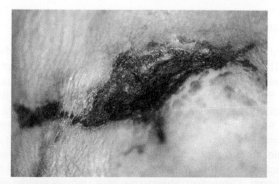

Fig. 2. Calciphylaxis. An eschar over the lateral thigh of a woman who self-administered excessive doses of vitamin D and calcium in the belief that she needed such doses for enhanced health. She developed deep ulcerative lesions over her thighs and buttocks, and some of the lesions evolved eschars such as this one. She died of infection because of compromise of her integument.

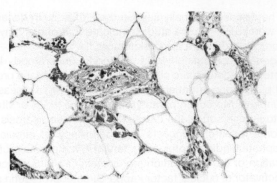

Fig. 3. Calciphylaxis. Calcium deposits within blood vessels of the subcutaneous fat. Irregular purple spicules of calcium are shown within vessel walls.

Treatment of calciphylaxis remains largely empiric because of its rarity, the incomplete knowledge with regard to its etiopathogenesis, and the absence of therapies showing clear-cut efficacy. Stopping possible offending agents (eg, calcium and vitamin D supplements) and adequate pain control are essential measures. When identified, hypercalcemia and hyperphosphatemia should be corrected to a target calcium × phosphate product less than 55 mg²/dL². The use of corticosteroids in calciphylaxis remains controversial.[17,19,34] Agents such as bisphosphonates, cinacalcet, and tissue plasminogen activator have been tried with mixed results.[35–38] Nonpharmacologic interventions like hemodialysis intensification with low-calcium dialysates, parathyroidectomy, and hyperbaric oxygen have also been used with variable outcomes.[23,39–41] Unless otherwise indicated, anticoagulation is not generally indicated. More recently, encouraging preliminary results have been obtained with intravenous administration of sodium thiosulfate (STS).[31,39,42–44] Although good response to STS is typically heralded by rapid improvement of the cutaneous pain, complete resolution of the skin lesions can take up to several months.[36,42] Possible complications of this therapy include the development of metabolic acidosis. However, the mortality of calciphylaxis commonly exceeds 50% and is usually caused by sepsis.[19,34,42] Therefore, aggressive wound care such as surgical debridement when necessary, and prompt antibiotic therapy for superinfected lesions are perhaps the most important therapeutic interventions.[17,39,40]

SEGMENTAL ARTERIAL MEDIOLYSIS

Segmental arterial mediolysis (SAM) is a rare noninflammatory arteriopathy of unknown cause.[45] This condition has been described in all age groups, but mainly affects adults and elderly individuals, with a slight male predominance. The disease is characterized by the occurrence of vacuolization of tissue in the outer portion of the media. This vacuolization leads to tearing and separation of the media from the adventitia (mediolysis). As the lesion progresses, the internal elastic lamina and the intima are destroyed, creating gaps that allow the blood-filled lumen to dissect into the adventitia. The blood then dissects the vessel wall through the media, presumably because of the action of hemodynamic forces, creating intramural hematomas and dissecting aneurysms. Dissecting aneurysms is a unique arterial lesion combining luminal stenosis with dilatation of the blood vessel diameter. Superimposed thrombosis and arterial rupture are frequently seen.

SAM mainly targets medium-sized arteries within the abdominal cavity. The aorta is almost never involved in SAM, but the celiac trunk, the superior and inferior mesenteric arteries, and their branches are involved in more than 80% of cases.[45] Less frequently, the renal, coronary, carotid, and intracranial arteries are affected.[46] The typical clinical picture consists of acute-onset abdominal pain; usually self-limited. Renal infarctions may prompt further evaluation in either SAM or FMD. Other manifestations of SAM include hematochezia, lumbar or flank pain, gross hematuria, acute coronary syndrome, pancreatitis, subarachnoid hemorrhage, and stroke.[47–49] Catastrophic presentations caused by arterial rupture, resulting in hemoperitoneum or retroperitoneal bleeding, occur in less than 30% of patients but are associated with high mortality.[50,51] In addition, SAM can also be subclinical and is sometimes identified incidentally when subjects are imaged for other reasons.[52]

In the absence of easily accessible tissue for biopsy, the diagnosis of SAM relies on identifying representative vascular imaging abnormalities (ie, angiography, CTA, and MRI/MRA) and excluding other entities. Angiographic findings comprise nonspecific arterial aneurysms, stenoses and occlusions, and the characteristic dissecting aneurysms (**Fig. 4**).[47,50,53] The differential diagnosis of SAM includes vasculitides (mainly PAN, Behçet disease, and TAK), mycotic aneurysm, and noninflammatory vasculopathies such as FMD, Ehlers-Danlos syndrome type IV, cystic adventitial artery disease, and cystic medial necrosis (eg, Marfan syndrome).[54,55] No serum or genetic biomarker is available for the diagnosis of SAM.

The treatment of SAM depends on the clinical manifestations. Many presentations resolve spontaneously without major consequences and can be managed conservatively. For cases of arterial rupture and hemorrhagic shock, either intravascular (eg, transarterial coil embolization) or surgical interventions are indicated depending on the gravity of the case.[56,57] Arterial instrumentation should be avoided whenever possible, because such procedures can lead to arterial dissections.

ANTIPHOSPHOLIPID SYNDROME

The APS is a condition characterized by thrombosis and pregnancy morbidity in the context of circulating antiphospholipid antibodies (aPL).[58] APS can affect all age groups in both genders, but is significantly more common in middle-aged women.

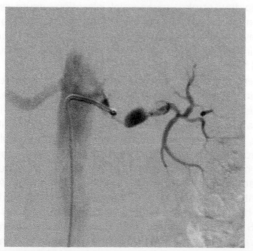

Fig. 4. SAM. Conventional angiography in a patient with SAM showing aneurysmal dilatation of the right renal artery. (*Courtesy of* Dr George Oliveira, Massachusetts General Hospital.)

The disorder may occur in isolation (ie, primary APS) or in the setting of systemic auto-immune diseases such as SLE.[59–61]

aPL are a heterogeneous group of immunoglobulins directed against anionic phospholipids or plasma proteins bound to anionic phospholipids (eg, β-2 glycoprotein I or prothrombin). On binding to their antigen, aPL trigger both the clotting and complement cascades and activate cell receptors (eg, apolipoprotein E receptor 2) on the surface of platelets, endothelial cells, and leucocytes.[59,62] Arterial and venous thromboses are the major features of the syndrome.[63] The most common vascular beds affected are the deep veins of the lower extremities, and the pulmonary, coronary, and intracranial circulation. In addition, several noncriteria clinical features have been described, including thrombocytopenia, hemolytic anemia, valvular heart disease, seizures, cognitive impairment, transverse myelitis, movement disorder (eg, chorea), brain white matter lesions, and renal and skin manifestations (discussed later).[63,64] An aPL-associated vasculopathy has also been described in association with the mammalian TORC (mTORC) pathway.[65] Some clinical data suggest that sirolimus (rapamycin), an inhibitor of the mTORC pathway, may have therapeutic utility in some APS cases, but this hypothesis requires confirmation. A small percentage of patients with APS develop diffuse alveolar hemorrhage either caused by capillaritis or bleeding diathesis (eg, antithrombin antibodies).[66–68] Leukocytoclastic vasculitis and responsiveness to the combination of rituximab and anticoagulation have been described in such cases.

APS skin manifestations such as livedo reticularis, livedoid vasculopathy (atrophie blanche), lower extremity ulcers, cutaneous necrosis, digital gangrene, and pseudo-vasculitic nodules and macules can be difficult to differentiate from PAN, ANCA-associated vasculitis, cryoglobulinemic vasculitis, and Henoch-Schönlein purpura.[64,69–72] The distinction between vasculitis and APS is of paramount importance given its therapeutic implications (ie, anticoagulation). aPL nephropathy, which comprises thrombotic microangiopathy and to a lesser extent membranous nephropathy, can represent a challenging differential diagnosis as well. Approximately 1% of patients with APS develop a particularly severe form of disease referred as catastrophic APS (CAPS).[63] Patients with CAPS present with systemic inflammatory response (eg, fever, tachycardia) and widespread macrovascular/microvascular clotting that may lead to encephalopathy, stroke, myocardial infraction, acute respiratory distress, pulmonary embolism, acute kidney injury, and intra-abdominal thrombosis.[68] The clinical picture then may resemble severe sepsis, thrombotic thrombocytopenia purpura, and disseminated intravascular coagulopathy. The mTORC pathway has also been implicated in CAPS.[65]

The key to differentiating APS from vasculitis relies on the presence of persistently circulating aPL (ie, anticardiolipins, anti–β-2 glycoprotein 1 antibodies, and lupus anticoagulant), and the histologic features of the different conditions. Although vasculitides show distinctive anatomopathologic abnormalities (eg, vascular wall fibrinoid necrosis, mural inflammation, immune complex deposition, and even vascular thrombosis as a result of inflammation), the characteristic finding of APS when it affects medium and small vessels is a bland thrombus with absent or minimal vascular or perivascular inflammation.[59] In addition, other serologic markers such as ANCA and cryoglobulins contribute importantly to the approach to diagnosis. The treatment of APS usually requires intravenous heparin followed by oral warfarin.[59] In addition to anticoagulation, patients with CAPS might benefit from high doses of corticosteroids and, at times, plasma exchanges and additional immunosuppression (eg, rituximab, cyclophosphamide).[68] Sirolimus has been proposed for patients with APS-associated vasculopathy in the kidneys and for those with CAPS, but this approach requires further testing.[65]

HYPEREOSINOPHILIC SYNDROME

Hypereosinophilic syndrome (HES) is a group of rare disorders mediated by eosinophil-driven end-organ damage. The diagnosis requires the presence of persistent eosinophilia (>1500 × 10⁹/L for 6 months) typically accompanied by eosinophilic infiltration of end organs.[73] Men are more commonly affected than women and the condition typically affects adults in the third to sixth decade of life.[74] A commonly encountered diagnostic challenge is distinguishing HES from conditions associated with hypereosinophilia, such as eosinophilic granulomatosis with polyangiitis (EGPA; formerly Churg-Strauss syndrome), sarcoidosis, systemic mastocytosis, and inflammatory bowel disease.[73] This article focuses on the differentiation between HES and EGPA, because these syndromes have many similar presenting features but differ markedly in their treatment.

HES can present with cardiovascular (58%), cutaneous (56%), neurologic (54%), pulmonary (49%), hepatic (30%), and gastrointestinal manifestations (14%), although frequencies of organ involvement differ considerably among series.[74,75] Both EGPA and HES can present with myocarditis, cardiomyopathy, pulmonary infiltrates, peripheral neuropathy, or erythematous skin lesions. Clinical characteristics that can help distinguish EGPA from HES include the presence of asthma and sinonasal disease such as sinusitis, allergic rhinitis, and nasal polyposis, which are present infrequently in HES.[75] In contrast, angioedema and splenomegaly are more common in HES. An important distinguishing feature between the two conditions is the presence of vasculitis, which is seen principally in EGPA. Therefore, skin lesions such as palpable purpura or vasculitic nodules suggest EGPA, although vasculitic lesions and ischemic lesions from arterial microthrombi have rarely been reported in HES.[76,77] Mononeuritis multiplex, which is most commonly caused by a vasculitic process, similarly suggests a diagnosis of EGPA, although mononeuritis multiplex has been reported in several patients with HES.[78]

Laboratory examinations can further aid in the diagnosis. Serologic testing for ANCA strongly suggests EGPA when positive, but ANCA are absent in approximately 50% of patients with EGPA. If HES is suspected, further testing to confirm the diagnosis and determine the subtype of HES is indicated. The myeloproliferative form of HES can be detected with examination of the bone marrow in addition to blood or bone marrow aspirate testing for FIP1L1/PDGFRA fusion, which is present in a subset of such patients.[79] In addition, flow cytometry may be able to detect lymphocytic variants of HES, which are driven by an overproduction of cytokines that coordinate eosinophil production.[80] Tissue biopsy is an important diagnostic modality when attempting to differentiate EGPA and HES. Because vasculitis is seen infrequently in HES, the presence of vasculitis on pathology, particularly in a patient with a history of asthma or sinonasal disease, strongly suggests the diagnosis of EGPA.

The treatment of HES varies by disease subtype. First-line therapy for patients with the FIP1L1/PDGFRA mutation is a tyrosine kinase inhibitor (such as imatinib).[79] Glucocorticoids are the mainstay of treatment of the lymphocytic variants of HES, with the addition of glucocorticoid sparing agents such as hydroxyurea, interferon alfa, or other chemotherapeutic agents as necessary.[75] Because treatment options differ considerably between HES and EGPA, distinguishing HES from EGPA and other eosinophilic disorders is of the utmost importance.

LYMPHOMATOID GRANULOMATOSIS

LMPG is a rare syndrome most commonly affecting the lungs that was described originally by Liebow and colleagues[81] in 1972. Most experts think that LMPG is a myeloproliferative B-cell disorder associated with Epstein-Barr virus (EBV) infection.[82,83] Men are affected preferentially (approximately 2:1) and although the condition can be seen at any age, onset is most commonly in the fourth to sixth decade of life.[81] Occurrences of the disease among individuals receiving immunosuppressant therapy[84,85] or in patients with other known underlying immunodeficiencies have been reported, but such cases comprise a minority of LMPG diagnoses.[86]

Pulmonary manifestations are the most common form of involvement, affecting approximately 60% to 90% of patients.[83] LMPG appears radiologically as bilateral infiltrates and nodules that can mimic several rheumatologic conditions, including granulomatosis with polyangiitis (GPA), EGPA, and sarcoidosis. Constitutional symptoms are often present. The skin or the nervous system is also involved in approximately one-third of patients.[87] Cutaneous manifestations are most typically nodules or nonspecific erythematous lesions. Neurologic manifestations include symptoms resulting from cerebral or cerebellar involvement, as well as cranial or peripheral neuropathies. Hepatomegaly or splenomegaly has been reported in a minority of patients.[84]

The diagnosis of LMPG is made histologically. Because LMPG is characterized by a polymorphic infiltrate that can affect arteries and veins in addition to parenchymal tissues, it is often difficult to distinguish from certain forms of primary vasculitis (eg, GPA). Although areas of necrosis are commonly seen within the parenchymal infiltrate, necrosis of the blood vessel wall (the sine qua non of a true vasculitis) is absent in LMPG.[88] Another differentiating feature of LMPG is the presence of large, atypical-appearing lymphoid cells thought to be a clonal B-cell population.[89] These cells typically express CD-20 and staining for the presence of EBV is positive in most cases. In some cases, differentiation from lymphoma can be challenging. Although macrophages and spindle-shaped histiocytes are present, palisading and well-formed granulomas are typically absent.[85] Thus, the granulomatosis portion of the LMPG name exaggerates the granulomatous features that are present in this condition.

LMPG carries significant mortality, ranging from 38% to 71%, and is generally thought to be a form of lymphoma.[83] Optimal treatment relies on the accurate differentiation of LMPG from vasculitis.

MALIGNANT ATROPHIC PAPULOSIS

Malignant atrophic papulosis (MAP), also known as Kohlmeier-Degos disease, is a vasculopathy that can mimic vasculitis affecting the brain, skin, and gastrointestinal tract. Described in 1941 by Kohlmeier[90] and a year later by Degos and colleagues,[91] it is a rare entity with fewer than 200 cases reported in the literature to date.[90–92] Although its cause remains unknown, the condition has been described as a familial autosomal dominant disorder as well as in association with autoimmune conditions such as dermatomyositis.[93,94] The hallmark of the disease are characteristic skin lesions that appear as papules (0.5–1 cm) with a white, atrophic center and an erythematous rim, most commonly on the trunk and extremities (**Fig. 5**). The skin lesions typically appear weeks to years before clinically apparent involvement of other organs.[94] In some cases the condition remains limited to the skin, leading some experts to suggest the term benign cutaneous Degos disease for this patient subset.[95] When internal organs are involved, the gastrointestinal tract (approximately 50% of patients) and the brain (approximately 20% of patients) are affected most commonly.[96] The lesions in these organs are similar in appearance to those in the skin and lead to ischemic complications such as stroke, bowel infarction, and hemorrhage. Mortality from ischemic complications is high: 50% of patients succumb to the disease within 2 to 3 years.[92]

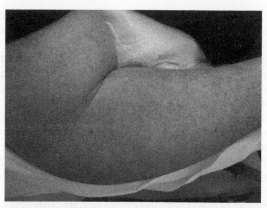

Fig. 5. Malignant atrophic papulosis. Skin lesions in a patient with malignant atrophic papulosis (Degos disease). Note the characteristic discreet porcelain papules with erythematous rim. These lesions are small and regular in appearance, differentiating them from atrophie blanche.

Because there are no diagnostic laboratory findings, the diagnosis is typically confirmed with skin biopsy. There are no diagnostic serologic or other laboratory findings. The pathology of MAP, regardless of the organ affected, consists of a thrombotic vasculopathy with intimal hyperplasia and thrombosis of small arteries. A lymphocytic vascular infiltrate can sometimes be seen, particularly early in the disease course.[97] Recently, C5b-9 deposition in the lesions, implicating complement in the pathogenesis, has been described.[98] Dysfunction of endothelial cells and fibrinolysis has also been implicated in MAP.[92]

Several therapies have been attempted in MAP but none has been widely successful to date, except in anecdotal cases. Success with antithrombotic agents and anticoagulants such as aspirin, dipyridamole, and heparin has been described in case reports.[96] Immunosuppression with glucocorticoids and cytotoxic agents have generally been ineffective.[96] Recent efforts have centered on inhibition of complement activation with eculizumab, a C5 inhibitor, but sustained remission remains elusive and most patients treated with eculizumab have succumbed to their illness.[99] New insights into disease pathophysiology are required for the development of more effective therapies.

REVERSIBLE CEREBRAL VASOCONSTRICTION SYNDROME

Reversible cerebral vasoconstriction syndrome (RCVS) is a heterogeneous group of conditions leading to vasoconstriction of arteries within the central nervous system (CNS). RCVS is one of the most common mimickers of primary and secondary CNS vasculitis. The condition is most commonly seen in clinical settings that serve as a trigger for vasospasm, such as the exposure to certain medications (pseudoephedrine, selective serotonin reuptake inhibitors, ergots, and many others) or during the postpartum period.[100] Women are affected more often than men and the average age at onset is in the third to fifth decade of life.[100,101]

The hallmark of RCVS is the sudden onset of severe headache, often described as thunderclap in nature. These types of headaches usually achieve their peak severity within a minute, raising concern about the possibility of subarachnoid hemorrhage, and can last for hours. Such headaches can recur over periods of days to weeks and are accompanied by neurologic deficits in approximately 40% of cases. Seizures have been reported in nearly 20% of patients. Vascular imaging shows diffuse vasoconstriction that cannot be distinguished from CNS vasculitis. The intensity of vasoconstriction in some RCVS cases is such that infarction (reported in up to 40% of cases), subarachnoid hemorrhage, and lobar intracerebral bleeding can occur.[101]

The combination of clinical features, cerebrospinal fluid (CSF) analysis, and imaging tests can help make the important distinction between RCVS and CNS vasculitis. Although the most common symptom of CNS vasculitis is headache, the quality is typically subacute to chronic and is less severe than the headache of RCVS. Lumbar puncture is normal in approximately 80% of patients with RCVS, in contrast with CNS vasculitis in which CSF pleocytosis or increased protein levels are seen in most patients.[102] Strokes can be observed in both conditions, but in RCVS the areas of infarction typically occur in the watershed regions. In contrast, ischemic lesions from CNS vasculitis can occur in both the cortex and the subcortex without a distinct vascular pattern.[102]

When medication-induced RCVS is suspected, the inciting agent should be removed immediately. There are no universally accepted treatment protocols for RCVS. However, several case series show good outcomes with nimodipine[103] or other calcium channel blockers.[101] A large retrospective series showed a trend toward worse outcomes with glucocorticoids, therefore currently there is no clear role for the use of steroids in RCVS, which underscores the importance of distinguishing between RCVS and CNS vasculitis.[101]

LIVEDOID VASCULOPATHY

Livedoid vasculopathy is a thrombotic condition affecting the small blood vessels of the skin; chiefly those of the lower extremities. Livedoid vasculopathy, sometimes also termed segmental hyalinizing vasculopathy, can be a primary condition or be associated with disorders such as inherited coagulopathies, the APS, Sneddon syndrome, venous insufficiency, varicosities, deep vein thrombosis, systemic lupus erythematosus, systemic sclerosis, rheumatoid arthritis, Sjögren syndrome, mixed connective tissue disease, or cancer.

The classic clinical lesion of livedoid vasculopathy is atrophie blanche: porcelain-colored scars sometimes dappled with small red points, occurring at the sites of ulcers (**Fig. 6**). Livedoid vasculopathy, which has a predilection for the tops of the feet, the perimalleolar areas, and the distal legs, often mimics medium vessel vasculitides such as polyarteritis nodosa, cutaneous polyarteritis nodosa, rheumatoid vasculitis, and the vasculitis associated with Sjögren syndrome. The typical skin lesions begin

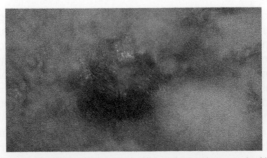

Fig. 6. Atrophie blanche. Porcelain-colored scarring on a background of hyperpigmentation (hemosiderin) in a patient with livedoid vasculopathy.

as tender erythematous nodules that then rapidly ulcerate and scar with atrophie blanche. The ulcers have an irregular shape and are extremely painful.

An adequate skin biopsy is required to make the diagnosis but multiple, repeated biopsies are discouraged because the biopsy sites can be slow to heal. Histopathologic examination of the lesions shows a thin and flattened epidermis. The superficial dermis shows segmental hyalinization of small vessels, endothelial swelling, and dilated capillaries with tortuous loops. Hemosiderin or extravasated red blood cells can be observed. Microthrombi are present in most cases. Although a perivascular lymphocytic infiltrate is a part of the morphologic picture, there is no damage to the blood vessel wall. Fibrinoid necrosis of the vessel wall, leukocytoclasis, and frank vasculitis are all absent in livedoid vasculopathy.

The pathophysiology of livedoid vasculopathy is not fully understood and the condition is likely not a single pathophysiologic entity but rather a final common pathway resulting from a variety of issues (often more than 1) that facilitate a hypercoagulable state. aPL are often present in this condition, as are other hypercoagulable risk factors including heritable factors (eg, the factor V Leiden mutation), functional or de facto protein C or S deficiency, the use of oral contraceptives, and smoking. A thorough review and evaluation for hypercoagulable risk factors should be undertaken when assessing patients for the possibility of livedoid vasculopathy.

A host of therapies, all generally designed to interrupt the tendency to coagulation, have been used in this condition. Therapies include baby aspirin, dipyridamole, low-molecular-weight heparin, Coumadin, and hydroxychloroquine.[104] Combinations of these agents are often used, and empiric approaches are typically required.

IMMUNOGLOBULIN G4–RELATED DISEASE

IgG4-RD, a fibroinflammatory condition that has emerged in recognition only in the past 10 years, is a subtle mimicker of multiple rheumatologic and malignant conditions, including the vasculitides.[105] In 2 important respects, IgG4-RD may even be not only a vasculitis mimic but a form of vasculitis. First, on a microscopic level, vasculotropism is a cardinal pathology feature of this disease. Obliterative phlebitis and (less often) obliterative arteritis are hallmark pathology manifestations of IgG4-RD. Second, IgG4-RD can also affect the aorta with a true aortitis, creating confusion with giant cell aortitis and other forms of inflammatory aortitis.[106,107] Thus, IgG4-RD is a common mimicker of small and medium vessel vasculitides, particularly GPA, but it can also cause a true vasculitis of large vessels, requiring distinction from GCA, among other vasculitides.

IgG4-RD was identified first in the pancreas among patients with sclerosing pancreatitis,[108] now termed type 1 IgG4-related autoimmune pancreatitis,[109] but in the past decade the disease has been described in almost every organ system (striated muscle and the brain being the 2 main exceptions). The organs affected most frequently by IgG4-RD include the pancreas, the major salivary glands, orbital tissue (particularly the lacrimal glands), the biliary tree, lymph nodes, and the retroperitoneum (ie, retroperitoneal fibrosis).

IgG4-RD is defined pathologically by several features that are remarkably consistent from organ to organ.[110] These features include a lymphoplasmacytic infiltrate with a disproportionate percentage of plasma cells staining for IgG4 (**Fig. 7**), a highly characteristic form of fibrosis known as storiform fibrosis, mild to moderate tissue eosinophilia, and the aforementioned obliterative phlebitis. Neither increased serum IgG4 concentrations nor increased numbers of IgG4+ plasma cells in tissue are sufficient to establish the diagnosis of IgG4-RD. Clinical correlation between the classic

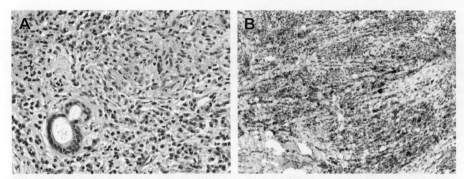

Fig. 7. IgG4-related disease: histopathology and immunopathology. Biopsy of a subglottic lesion affecting a 70-year-old woman who also had large vessel imaging that was diagnostic of aortitis. The subglottic lesion mimicked GPA. The patient's antineutrophil cytoplasmic antibody assay was negative, but her serum IgG4 concentration was increased to 3 times the upper limit of normal. (A) Histopathology. Subglottic lesion showing a lymphoplasmacytic infiltrate and a swirling, storiform pattern of fibrosis (hematoxylin-eosin stain, magnification 400×). (B) Immunopathology. Immunostain for IgG4, showing more than 50 IgG4+ plasma cells (brown-staining cells) per high-power field (magnification 400×).

histopathologic findings (lymphoplasmacytic tissue infiltrate, storiform fibrosis, obliterative phlebitis) and rigorous clinicopathologic correlation are required.

The propensity of IgG4-RD to affect multiple organs and its ability to affect the orbits, lungs, kidneys, and pachymeninges also make it a particularly effective mimicker of GPA. IgG4-RD can cause proptosis through involvement of several orbital structures, including the lacrimal gland, extraocular muscles, and retrobulbar mass lesions that are independent of these structures. Scleritis and involvement of the nasolacrimal duct, both common features of GPA, have also been reported in IgG4-RD.[111]

The lung is the site of the most protean involvement of IgG4-RD. The disease has a tendency to affect the bronchovascular bundle, leading to thickening of the airways on cross-sectional imaging. Mass pulmonary lesions can also be observed in IgG4-RD, imitating malignant lesions or the nodules of GPA. Ground-glass infiltrates and interstitial fibrosis are also seen, mimicking either alveolar hemorrhage or the interstitial lung disease sometimes associated with ANCA-associated vasculitis, particularly cases associated with antimyeloperoxidase ANCA. Subglottic stenosis, other types of large airway involvement, and extensive pleural disease are also known to occur in IgG4-RD.

The typical renal manifestation of IgG4-RD is tubulointerstitial nephritis, presenting chiefly with renal dysfunction and white blood cells in the urine. A membranous glomerulonephropathy (GN) has also been reported to occur in this disease. The IgG4-related membranous GN is clearly a condition distinct from idiopathic membranous GN, which is associated with autoantibodies (usually IgG4) directed against the PLA2 receptor. In addition, IgG4-RD is an important cause of idiopathic hypertrophic pachymeningitis and rivals GPA as a cause of that condition.[112]

The first line of therapy for IgG4-RD is generally glucocorticoids. Most patients with IgG4-RD respond to glucocorticoids and in many patients the response is striking, reminiscent of the types of response observed in GCA and polymyalgia rheumatica following the institution of steroids. However, most patients, particularly those with multiorgan disease at baseline, relapse during or after glucocorticoid tapers. Moreover, because IgG4-RD tends to target middle-aged to elderly patients and to affect the pancreas, lengthy courses of glucocorticoids are generally tolerated poorly. Among patients whose disease is refractory to glucocorticoids or to glucocorticoid tapers or whose comorbidities suggest that glucocorticoids will be tolerated poorly, B-cell depletion with rituximab seems to be an excellent therapy (Carruthers MN, Topazian MD, Khosroshahi A, et al. Rituximab for IgG4-related disease: a prospective, open-label trial. Submitted for publication).[113]

REFERENCES

1. Slovut DP, Olin JW. Fibromuscular dysplasia. N Engl J Med 2004;350(18): 1862–71.
2. Persu A, Giavarini A, Touze E, et al. European consensus on the diagnosis and management of fibromuscular dysplasia. J Hypertens 2014;32(7):1367–78.
3. Olin JW, Froehlich J, Gu X, et al. The United States Registry for Fibromuscular Dysplasia: results in the first 447 patients. Circulation 2012;125(25):3182–90.
4. McKenzie GA, Oderich GS, Kawashima A, et al. Renal artery fibromuscular dysplasia in 2,640 renal donor subjects: a CT angiography analysis. J Vasc Interv Radiol 2013;24(10):1477–80.
5. Olin JW, Gornik HL, Bacharach JM, et al. Fibromuscular dysplasia: state of the science and critical unanswered questions: a scientific statement from the American Heart Association. Circulation 2014;129(9):1048–78.
6. Savard S, Steichen O, Azarine A, et al. Association between 2 angiographic subtypes of renal artery fibromuscular dysplasia and clinical characteristics. Circulation 2012;126(25):3062–9.
7. Pannier-Moreau I, Grimbert P, Fiquet-Kempf B, et al. Possible familial origin of multifocal renal artery fibromuscular dysplasia. J Hypertens 1997;15(12 Pt 2): 1797–801.
8. Mettinger KL, Ericson K. Fibromuscular dysplasia and the brain. I. Observations on angiographic, clinical and genetic characteristics. Stroke 1982;13(1): 46–52.
9. Miller DJ, Marin H, Aho T, et al. Fibromuscular dysplasia unraveled: the pulsation-induced microtrauma and reactive hyperplasia theory. Med Hypotheses 2014;83(1):21–4.
10. Tweet MS, Hayes SN, Pitta SR, et al. Clinical features, management, and prognosis of spontaneous coronary artery dissection. Circulation 2012;126(5): 579–88.
11. Kim ES, Olin JW, Froehlich JB, et al. Clinical manifestations of fibromuscular dysplasia vary by patient sex: a report of the United States registry for fibromuscular dysplasia. J Am Coll Cardiol 2013;62(21):2026–8.
12. Cloft HJ, Kallmes DF, Kallmes MH, et al. Prevalence of cerebral aneurysms in patients with fibromuscular dysplasia: a reassessment. J Neurosurg 1998; 88(3):436–40.
13. Hagg A, Lorelius LE, Morlin C, et al. Percutaneous transluminal renal artery dilatation for fibromuscular dysplasia with special reference to the acute effects on the renin-angiotensin-aldosterone-system and blood pressure. Acta Med Scand Suppl 1985;693:93–6.
14. Trinquart L, Mounier-Vehier C, Sapoval M, et al. Efficacy of revascularization for renal artery stenosis caused by fibromuscular dysplasia: a systematic review and meta-analysis. Hypertension 2010;56(3):525–32.
15. Brott TG, Halperin JL, Abbara S, et al. 2011 ASA/ACCF/AHA/AANN/AANS/ACR/ ASNR/CNS/SAIP/SCAI/SIR/SNIS/SVM/SVS guideline on the management of

patients with extracranial carotid and vertebral artery disease: executive summary. A report of the American College of Cardiology Foundation/American Heart Association Task Force on Practice Guidelines, and the American Stroke Association, American Association of Neuroscience Nurses, American Association of Neurological Surgeons, American College of Radiology, American Society of Neuroradiology, Congress of Neurological Surgeons, Society of Atherosclerosis Imaging and Prevention, Society for Cardiovascular Angiography and Interventions, Society of Interventional Radiology, Society of Neurointerventional Surgery, Society for Vascular Medicine, and Society for Vascular Surgery. Circulation 2011;124(4):489–532.

16. Kennedy F, Lanfranconi S, Hicks C, et al. Antiplatelets vs anticoagulation for dissection: CADISS nonrandomized arm and meta-analysis. Neurology 2012; 79(7):686–9.

17. Weenig RH, Sewell LD, Davis MD, et al. Calciphylaxis: natural history, risk factor analysis, and outcome. J Am Acad Dermatol 2007;56(4):569–79.

18. Angelis M, Wong LL, Myers SA, et al. Calciphylaxis in patients on hemodialysis: a prevalence study. Surgery 1997;122(6):1083–9 [discussion: 1089–90].

19. Nigwekar SU, Wolf M, Sterns RH, et al. Calciphylaxis from nonuremic causes: a systematic review. Clin J Am Soc Nephrol 2008;3(4):1139–43.

20. Hayashi M, Takamatsu I, Kanno Y, et al. A case-control study of calciphylaxis in Japanese end-stage renal disease patients. Nephrol Dial Transplant 2012; 27(4):1580–4.

21. Wong JJ, Laumann A, Martinez M. Calciphylaxis and antiphospholipid antibody syndrome. J Am Acad Dermatol 2000;42(5 Pt 1):849.

22. Lee JL, Naguwa SM, Cheema G, et al. Recognizing calcific uremic arteriolopathy in autoimmune disease: an emerging mimicker of vasculitis. Autoimmun Rev 2008;7(8):638–43.

23. Arch-Ferrer JE, Beenken SW, Rue LW, et al. Therapy for calciphylaxis: an outcome analysis. Surgery 2003;134(6):941–4 [discussion: 944–5].

24. Janigan DT, Hirsch DJ, Klassen GA, et al. Calcified subcutaneous arterioles with infarcts of the subcutis and skin ("calciphylaxis") in chronic renal failure. Am J Kidney Dis 2000;35(4):588–97.

25. Selye H, Gabbiani G, Strebel R. Sensitization to calciphylaxis by endogenous parathyroid hormone. Endocrinology 1962;71:554–8.

26. Schafer C, Heiss A, Schwarz A, et al. The serum protein alpha 2-Heremans-Schmid glycoprotein/fetuin-A is a systemically acting inhibitor of ectopic calcification. J Clin Invest 2003;112(3):357–66.

27. Luo G, Ducy P, McKee MD, et al. Spontaneous calcification of arteries and cartilage in mice lacking matrix GLA protein. Nature 1997;386(6620):78–81.

28. Mehta RL, Scott G, Sloand JA, et al. Skin necrosis associated with acquired protein C deficiency in patients with renal failure and calciphylaxis. Am J Med 1990;88(3):252–7.

29. Ma YL, Cain RL, Halladay DL, et al. Catabolic effects of continuous human PTH (1–38) in vivo is associated with sustained stimulation of RANKL and inhibition of osteoprotegerin and gene-associated bone formation. Endocrinology 2001;142(9):4047–54.

30. Edelstein CL, Wickham MK, Kirby PA. Systemic calciphylaxis presenting as a painful, proximal myopathy. Postgrad Med J 1992;68(797):209–11.

31. Araya CE, Fennell RS, Neiberger RE, et al. Sodium thiosulfate treatment for calcific uremic arteriolopathy in children and young adults. Clin J Am Soc Nephrol 2006;1(6):1161–6.

32. O'Neil B, Southwick AW. Three cases of penile calciphylaxis: diagnosis, treatment strategies, and the role of sodium thiosulfate. Urology 2012;80(1):5–8.
33. Norris B, Vaysman V, Line BR. Bone scintigraphy of calciphylaxis: a syndrome of vascular calcification and skin necrosis. Clin Nucl Med 2005;30(11):725–7.
34. Fine A, Zacharias J. Calciphylaxis is usually non-ulcerating: risk factors, outcome and therapy. Kidney Int 2002;61(6):2210–7.
35. Robinson MR, Augustine JJ, Korman NJ. Cinacalcet for the treatment of calciphylaxis. Arch Dermatol 2007;143(2):152–4
36. Salmhofer H, Franzen M, Hitzl W, et al. Multi-modal treatment of calciphylaxis with sodium-thiosulfate, cinacalcet and sevelamer including long-term data. Kidney Blood Press Res 2013;37(4–5):346–59.
37. Schliep S, Schuler G, Kiesewetter F. Successful treatment of calciphylaxis with pamidronate. Eur J Dermatol 2008;18(5):554–6.
38. el-Azhary RA, Arthur AK, Davis MD, et al. Retrospective analysis of tissue plasminogen activator as an adjuvant treatment for calciphylaxis. JAMA Dermatol 2013;149(1):63–7.
39. Baldwin C, Farah M, Leung M, et al. Multi-intervention management of calciphylaxis: a report of 7 cases. Am J Kidney Dis 2011;58(6):988–91.
40. Girotto JA, Harmon JW, Ratner LE, et al. Parathyroidectomy promotes wound healing and prolongs survival in patients with calciphylaxis from secondary hyperparathyroidism. Surgery 2001;130(4):645–50 [discussion: 650–1].
41. Alikadic N, Kovac D, Krasna M, et al. Review of calciphylaxis and treatment of a severe case after kidney transplantation with iloprost in combination with hyperbaric oxygen and cultured autologous fibrin-based skin substitutes. Clin Transplant 2009;23(6):968–74.
42. Noureddine L, Landis M, Patel N, et al. Efficacy of sodium thiosulfate for the treatment for calciphylaxis. Clin Nephrol 2011;75(6):485–90.
43. Auriemma M, Carbone A, Di Liberato L, et al. Treatment of cutaneous calciphylaxis with sodium thiosulfate: two case reports and a review of the literature. Am J Clin Dermatol 2011;12(5):339–46.
44. Fernandes C, Maynard B, Hanna D. Successful treatment of calciphylaxis with intravenous sodium thiosulfate in a nonuremic patient: case report and review of therapy side effects. J Cutan Med Surg 2014;18:1–5.
45. Pillai AK, Iqbal SI, Liu RW, et al. Segmental arterial mediolysis. Cardiovasc Intervent Radiol 2014;37(3):604–12.
46. Shenouda M, Riga C, Naji Y, et al. Segmental arterial mediolysis: a systematic review of 85 cases. Ann Vasc Surg 2014;28(1):269–77.
47. Kalva SP, Somarouthu B, Jaff MR, et al. Segmental arterial mediolysis: clinical and imaging features at presentation and during follow-up. J Vasc Interv Radiol 2011;22(10):1380–7.
48. Matsuda R, Hironaka Y, Takeshima Y, et al. Subarachnoid hemorrhage in a case of segmental arterial mediolysis with coexisting intracranial and intraabdominal aneurysms. J Neurosurg 2012;116(5):948–51.
49. Leu HJ. Cerebrovascular accidents resulting from segmental mediolytic arteriopathy of the cerebral arteries in young adults. Cardiovasc Surg 1994;2(3):350–3.
50. Slavin RE. Segmental arterial mediolysis: course, sequelae, prognosis, and pathologic-radiologic correlation. Cardiovasc Pathol 2009;18(6):352–60.
51. Phillips CK, Lepor H. Spontaneous retroperitoneal hemorrhage caused by segmental arterial mediolysis. Rev Urol 2006;8(1):36–40.
52. Hirakawa E, Inada K, Tsuji K. Asymptomatic dissecting aneurysm of the coeliac artery: a variant of segmental arterial mediolysis. Histopathology 2005;47(5):544–6.

53. Michael M, Widmer U, Wildermuth S, et al. Segmental arterial mediolysis: CTA findings at presentation and follow-up. AJR Am J Roentgenol 2006;187(6):1463–9.
54. Baker-LePain JC, Stone DH, Mattis AN, et al. Clinical diagnosis of segmental arterial mediolysis: differentiation from vasculitis and other mimics. Arthritis Care Res (Hoboken) 2010;62(11):1655–60.
55. Chan RJ, Goodman TA, Aretz TH, et al. Segmental mediolytic arteriopathy of the splenic and hepatic arteries mimicking systemic necrotizing vasculitis. Arthritis Rheum 1998;41(5):935–8.
56. Shimohira M, Ogino H, Sasaki S, et al. Transcatheter arterial embolization for segmental arterial mediolysis. J Endovasc Ther 2008;15(4):493–7.
57. Obara H, Matsumoto K, Narimatsu Y, et al. Reconstructive surgery for segmental arterial mediolysis involving both the internal carotid artery and visceral arteries. J Vasc Surg 2006;43(3):623–6.
58. Miyakis S, Lockshin MD, Atsumi T, et al. International consensus statement on an update of the classification criteria for definite antiphospholipid syndrome (APS). J Thromb Haemost 2006;4(2):295–306.
59. Ruiz-Irastorza G, Crowther M, Branch W, et al. Antiphospholipid syndrome. Lancet 2010;376(9751):1498–509.
60. Springer J, Villa-Forte A. Thrombosis in vasculitis. Curr Opin Rheumatol 2013; 25(1):19–25.
61. Gaffo AL. Thrombosis in vasculitis. Best Pract Res Clin Rheumatol 2013;27(1): 57–67.
62. Giannakopoulos B, Krilis SA. The pathogenesis of the antiphospholipid syndrome. N Engl J Med 2013;368(11):1033–44.
63. Cervera R, Serrano R, Pons-Estel GJ, et al. Morbidity and mortality in the antiphospholipid syndrome during a 10-year period: a multicentre prospective study of 1000 patients. Ann Rheum Dis 2014. [Epub ahead of print].
64. Erkan D, Vega J, Ramon G, et al. A pilot open-label phase II trial of rituximab for non-criteria manifestations of antiphospholipid syndrome. Arthritis Rheum 2013; 65(2):464–71.
65. Canaud G, Bienaime F, Tabarin F, et al. Inhibition of the mTORC pathway in the antiphospholipid syndrome. N Engl J Med 2014;371(4):303–12.
66. Cartin-Ceba R, Peikert T, Ashrani A, et al. Primary antiphospholipid syndrome-associated diffuse alveolar hemorrhage. Arthritis Care Res (Hoboken) 2014; 66(2):301–10.
67. Asherson RA, Cervera R, Wells AU. Diffuse alveolar hemorrhage: a nonthrombotic antiphospholipid lung syndrome? Semin Arthritis Rheum 2005;35(3):138–42.
68. Cervera R. Update on the diagnosis, treatment, and prognosis of the catastrophic antiphospholipid syndrome. Curr Rheumatol Rep 2010;12(1):70–6.
69. Gonzalez ME, Kahn P, Price HN, et al. Retiform purpura and digital gangrene secondary to antiphospholipid syndrome successfully treated with sildenafil. Arch Dermatol 2011;147(2):164–7.
70. Reyes E, Alarcon-Segovia D. Leg ulcers in the primary antiphospholipid syndrome. Report of a case with a peculiar proliferative small vessel vasculopathy. Clin Exp Rheumatol 1991;9(1):63–6.
71. Asherson RA, Jacobelli S, Rosenberg H, et al. Skin nodules and macules resembling vasculitis in the antiphospholipid syndrome–a report of two cases. Clin Exp Dermatol 1992;17(4):266–9.
72. Frances C, Niang S, Laffitte E, et al. Dermatologic manifestations of the antiphospholipid syndrome: two hundred consecutive cases. Arthritis Rheum 2005;52(6):1785–93.

73. Klion AD, Bochner BS, Gleich GJ, et al. Approaches to the treatment of hyper-eosinophilic syndromes: a workshop summary report. J Allergy Clin Immunol 2006;117(6):1292–302.
74. Sheikh J, Weller PF. Clinical overview of hypereosinophilic syndromes. Immunol Allergy Clin North Am 2007;27(3):333–55.
75. Ogbogu PU, Bochner BS, Butterfield JH, et al. Hypereosinophilic syndrome: a multicenter, retrospective analysis of clinical characteristics and response to therapy. J Allergy Clin Immunol 2009;124(6):1319 25.e3.
76. Weller PF, Bubley GJ. The idiopathic hypereosinophilic syndrome. Blood 1994; 83(10):2759–79.
77. Hayashi M, Kawaguchi M, Mitsuhashi Y, et al. Case of hypereosinophilic syndrome with cutaneous necrotizing vasculitis. J Dermatol 2008;35(4):229–33.
78. Moore PM, Harley JB, Fauci AS. Neurologic dysfunction in the idiopathic hyper-eosinophilic syndrome. Ann Intern Med 1985;102(1):109–14.
79. Cools J, DeAngelo DJ, Gotlib J, et al. A tyrosine kinase created by fusion of the PDGFRA and FIP1L1 genes as a therapeutic target of imatinib in idiopathic hypereosinophilic syndrome. N Engl J Med 2003;348(13):1201–14.
80. Simon HU, Plotz SG, Dummer R, et al. Abnormal clones of T cells producing interleukin-5 in idiopathic eosinophilia. N Engl J Med 1999;341(15):1112–20.
81. Liebow AA, Carrington CR, Friedman PJ. Lymphomatoid granulomatosis. Hum Pathol 1972;3(4):457–558.
82. Guinee D Jr, Jaffe E, Kingma D, et al. Pulmonary lymphomatoid granulomatosis. Evidence for a proliferation of Epstein-Barr virus infected B-lymphocytes with a prominent T-cell component and vasculitis. Am J Surg Pathol 1994;18(8): 753–64.
83. Katzenstein AL, Doxtader E, Narendra S. Lymphomatoid granulomatosis: insights gained over 4 decades. Am J Surg Pathol 2010;34(12):e35–48.
84. Joseph R, Chacko B, Manipadam MT, et al. Pulmonary lymphomatoid granulo-matosis in a renal allograft recipient. Transpl Infect Dis 2008;10(1):52–5.
85. Katherine Martin L, Porcu P, Baiocchi RA, et al. Primary central nervous system lymphomatoid granulomatosis in a patient receiving azathioprine therapy. Clin Adv Hematol Oncol 2009;7(1):65–8.
86. Sebire NJ, Haselden S, Malone M, et al. Isolated EBV lymphoproliferative disease in a child with Wiskott-Aldrich syndrome manifesting as cutaneous lymphomatoid granulomatosis and responsive to anti-CD20 immunotherapy. J Clin Pathol 2003;56(7):555–7.
87. Katzenstein AL, Carrington CB, Liebow AA. Lymphomatoid granulomatosis: a clinicopathologic study of 152 cases. Cancer 1979;43(1):360–73.
88. Koss MN, Hochholzer L, Langloss JM, et al. Lymphomatoid granulomatosis: a clinicopathologic study of 42 patients. Pathology 1986;18(3):283–8.
89. Jaffe ES, Wilson WH. Lymphomatoid granulomatosis: pathogenesis, pathology and clinical implications. Cancer Surv 1997;30:233–48.
90. Kohlmeier W. Multiple Hautnekrosen bei Thrombangitis obliterans. Arch Dermatol Syph (Wien) 1941;181:783–92.
91. Degos R, Delort J, Tricot R. Dermatite papulosqameuse atrophiante. Bull Soc Fr Dermatol Syphiligr 1942;49:148–50.
92. Theodoridis A, Makrantonaki E, Zouboulis CC. Malignant atrophic papulosis (Kohlmeier-Degos disease) - a review. Orphanet J Rare Dis 2013;8:10.
93. Katz SK, Mudd LJ, Roenigk HH Jr. Malignant atrophic papulosis (Degos' disease) involving three generations of a family. J Am Acad Dermatol 1997;37(3 Pt 1): 480–4.

94. Burgin S, Stone JH, Shenoy-Bhangle AS, et al. Case records of the Massachusetts General Hospital. Case 18-2014. A 32-year-old man with a rash, myalgia, and weakness. N Engl J Med 2014;370(24):2327–37.

95. Heymann WR. Degos disease: considerations for reclassification. J Am Acad Dermatol 2009;61(3):505–6.

96. Scheinfeld N. Malignant atrophic papulosis. Clin Exp Dermatol 2007;32(5): 483–7.

97. Su WP, Schroeter AL, Lee DA, et al. Clinical and histologic findings in Degos' syndrome (malignant atrophic papulosis). Cutis 1985;35(2):131–8.

98. Magro CM, Poe JC, Kim C, et al. Degos disease: a C5b-9/interferon-alpha-mediated endotheliopathy syndrome. Am J Clin Pathol 2011;135(4):599–610.

99. Magro CM, Wang X, Garrett-Bakelman F, et al. The effects of Eculizumab on the pathology of malignant atrophic papulosis. Orphanet J Rare Dis 2013;8:185.

100. Calabrese LH, Dodick DW, Schwedt TJ, et al. Narrative review: reversible cerebral vasoconstriction syndromes. Ann Intern Med 2007;146(1):34–44.

101. Singhal AB, Hajj-Ali RA, Topcuoglu MA, et al. Reversible cerebral vasoconstriction syndromes: analysis of 139 cases. Arch Neurol 2011;68(8):1005–12.

102. Salvarani C, Brown RD Jr, Calamia KT, et al. Primary central nervous system vasculitis: analysis of 101 patients. Ann Neurol 2007;62(5):442–51.

103. Ducros A, Boukobza M, Porcher R, et al. The clinical and radiological spectrum of reversible cerebral vasoconstriction syndrome. A prospective series of 67 patients. Brain 2007;130(Pt 12):3091–101.

104. Callen JP. Livedoid vasculopathy: what it is and how the patient should be evaluated and treated. Arch Dermatol 2006;142(11):1481–2.

105. Stone JH, Zen Y, Deshpande V. IgG4-related disease. N Engl J Med 2012; 366(6):539–51.

106. Stone JH, Khosroshahi A, Hilgenberg A, et al. IgG4-related systemic disease and lymphoplasmacytic aortitis. Arthritis Rheum 2009;60(10):3139–45.

107. Stone JH, Khosroshahi A, Deshpande V, et al. IgG4-related systemic disease accounts for a significant proportion of thoracic lymphoplasmacytic aortitis cases. Arthritis Care Res (Hoboken) 2010;62(3):316–22.

108. Kamisawa T, Egawa N, Nakajima H. Autoimmune pancreatitis is a systemic autoimmune disease. Am J Gastroenterol 2003;98(12):2811–2.

109. Stone JH, Khosroshahi A, Deshpande V, et al. Recommendations for the nomenclature of IgG4-related disease and its individual organ system manifestations. Arthritis Rheum 2012;64(10):3061–7.

110. Deshpande V, Zen Y, Chan JK, et al. Consensus statement on the pathology of IgG4-related disease. Mod Pathol 2012;25(9):1181–92.

111. Wallace ZS, Deshpande V, Stone JH. Ophthalmic manifestations of IgG4-related disease: single-center experience and literature review. Semin Arthritis Rheum 2014;43(6):806–17.

112. Wallace ZS, Carruthers MN, Khosroshahi A, et al. IgG4-related disease and hypertrophic pachymeningitis. Medicine 2013;92(4):206–16.

113. Khosroshahi A, Carruthers MN, Deshpande V, et al. Rituximab for the treatment of IgG4-related disease: lessons from 10 consecutive patients. Medicine 2012; 91(1):57–66.

Index

Note: Page numbers of article titles are in **boldface** type.

A

ANCA vasculitis. *See* Antineutrophil cytoplasmic antibody–associated (ANCA) vasculitis
Angiography
    in PACNS diagnosis, 53–54
Antineutrophil cytoplasmic antibody
    correlation with disease activity, 4
    detection of, 2–3
    in EGPA, 13
    measurements of, 4
    specificity of
        implications of, 3–4
Antineutrophil cytoplasmic antibody (ANCA)–associated vasculitis, **1–19**
    APS and, 114–115
    classification of, 2
    comorbidities of
        management of, 11–12
    EGPA, 12–14. *See also* Eosinophilic granulomatosis with polyangiitis (EGPA)
    future considerations for, 12
    introduction, 1–2
    terminology related to, 2
    tissue biopsy in, 4–5
    treatment of, 5–11
        historical perspective, 5
        induction therapy in, 8–9
        maintenance therapy in, 9–11
        principles of, 5–7
Antiphospholipid antibodies
    APS and
        in systemic vasculitis, 114–118
    vasculitis in APS and, 110–111
Antiphospholipid syndrome (APS)
    mimicking primary systemic vasculitis, 147–148
    vasculitis in, **109–123**
        antiphospholipid antibodies and, 110–111, 114–118. *See also specific types*
        case reports of, 113–114
        future considerations in, 118
        introduction, 109–110
        manifestations of, 111–114
Apheresis
    in cryoglobulinemia management, 102
APS. *See* Antiphospholipid syndrome (APS)

Rheum Dis Clin N Am 41 (2015) 161–166
http://dx.doi.org/10.1016/S0889-857X(14)00116-1
0889-857X/15/$ – see front matter © 2015 Elsevier Inc. All rights reserved.

rheumatic.theclinics.com

Moving?

Make sure your subscription moves with you!

To notify us of your new address, find your **Clinics Account Number** (located on your mailing label above your name), and contact customer service at:

Email: journalscustomerservice-usa@elsevier.com

800-654-2452 (subscribers in the U.S. & Canada)
314-447-8871 (subscribers outside of the U.S. & Canada)

Fax number: 314-447-8029

Elsevier Health Sciences Division
Subscription Customer Service
3251 Riverport Lane
Maryland Heights, MO 63043

*To ensure uninterrupted delivery of your subscription, please notify us at least 4 weeks in advance of move.

Printed and bound by CPI Group (UK) Ltd, Croydon, CR0 4YY

03/10/2024

01040495-0014